Michel Montignac

The french
GI Diet

100 Low Carb Recipes

EDITIONS
Alpen

Exclusive copyrights:
©Alpen Éditions
9, avenue Albert II
98000 Monaco
Tel: +377 97 77 62 10
Fax: +377 97 77 62 11
web: www.alpen.mc

Printed in Italy
ISBN: 978-2-35934-040-2

Michel Montignac

The french
GI Diet

100 Low Carb Recipes

EDITIONS
Alpen

Contents

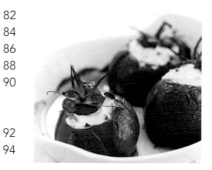

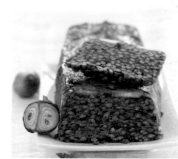

ENTREES

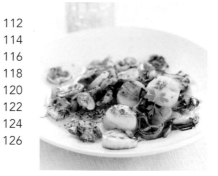

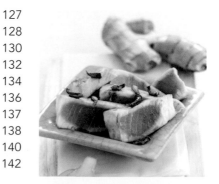

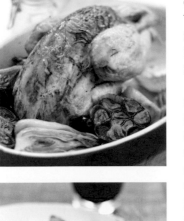

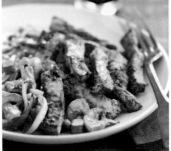

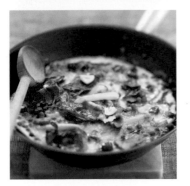

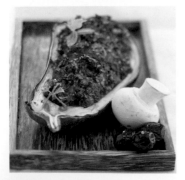

OTHERS

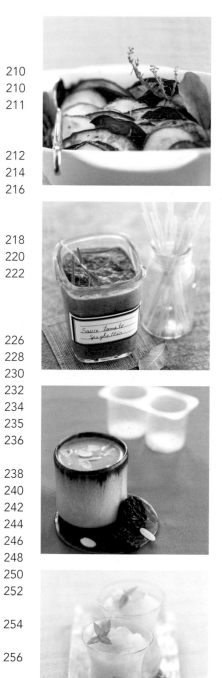

DESSERTS

Introduction

This recipe book is the second in a series launched at the beginning of the 1990's[1]. It proposes more than 100 new, illustrated recipes.

Like the earlier books, it in intended for all followers of the Montignac method, who will find in this work an additional field of application of the nutritional philosophy they follow.

It is also especially indicated for all those who wish to discover the principles of this method by getting started with practical work rather than studying the theory.

But this book is also for everyone, and especially women, who want to cook or start cooking again without complicating their lives at the same time. These recipes are simple, practical, gourmet and healthy.

• They are simple, since they involve basic culinary principles and, with few exceptions, anyone can make them, even beginners.

• They are easy because most of their ingredients are common and available everywhere. In addition, they do not require sophisticated material or utensils. The most elementary equipment is more than sufficient.

• They are gourmet, meaning they are primarily inspired by Provencal, or more generally Mediterranean cuisine, where sensory, olfactory, taste and visual pleasures are omnipresent.

• Lastly, these recipes are healthy since they comply with the principles of the Montignac method, which scientific studies (namely those of Professor Dumesnil[2]) have demonstrated that this nutritional approach helps prevent metabolic pathologies (obesity, diabetes, and cardio-vascular risk factors).

The first part of the book deals with a review of the Montignac method principles. Reading of this summary may serve as a good refresher for everyone who discovered the Montignac method years ago and who can use this book as an opportunity to update their knowledge. Since this method has not ceased to progress and to improve since its debut in 1986. If you are a long time follower, you should know that the idea of dissociation completely disappeared from the method starting at the beginning of the 1990's, and its mainstay is now the concept of the glycemic index.

If you are just discovering the Montignac method, an attentive reading of this summary will serve as a good initiation. You can always learn more by reading more specialized works[3].

The second part of the book includes nine weeks of examples of daily menus, integrating the book's recipes. You will also find a certain number of tips for using these menus like how to carry out the recipes.

The third part contains the essential part of this work: 100 illustrated recipes which I have the pleasure of proposing to you.

I hope you enjoy both making these recipes and eating the results.

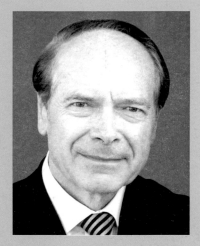

1. Michel Montignac, *The Montignac Diet Cookbook*, Alpen Editions, 2010.

Also available on the website shop: www.montignac-shop.com.

2. Dumesnil J.-G., *"Effect of a low glycemic index-low fat-high protein diet (Montignac) on the atherogenic metabolic risk profile of abdominally obese men"* in British Journal of Nutrition, November 2001.

3. Michel Montignac, *Eat Yourself Slim*, Alpen Editions, 2010.

Michel Montignac, *Glycemic Index Diet*, Alpen Editions, 2010.

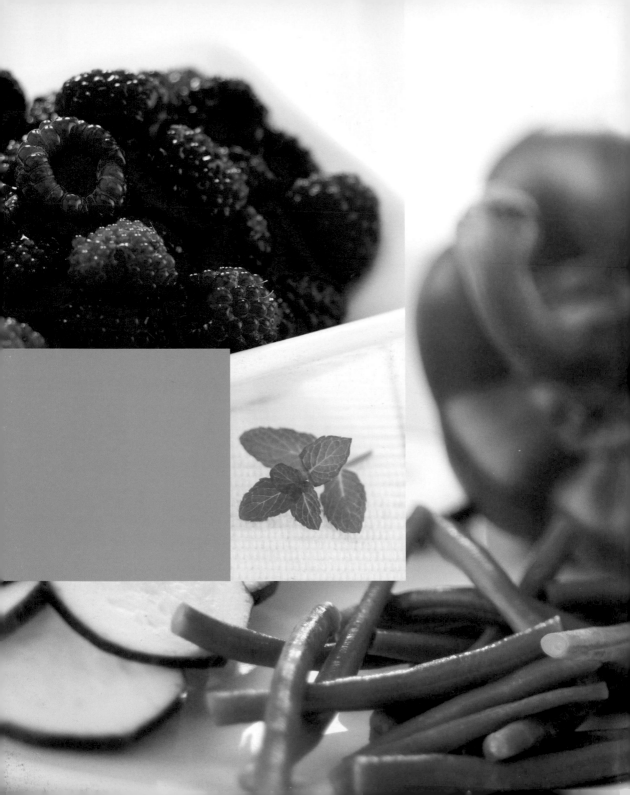

WHAT IS THE
MONTIGNAC
METHOD?

The Montignac method is a weight loss and maintenance program where the basic principle is a good selection of foods. It is not a diet, since it does not involve limiting quantities. It is a nutritional philosophy, a real lifestyle whose main goal is better health.

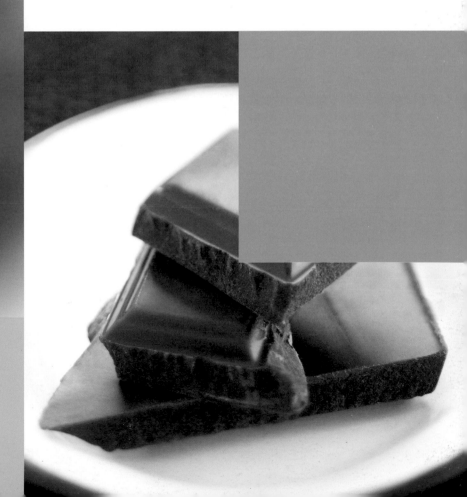

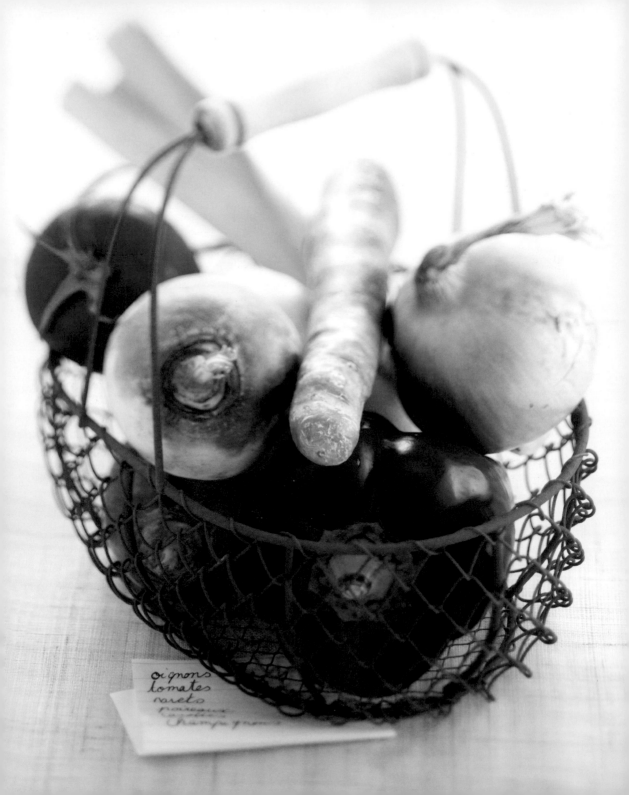

oignons
tomates
navets
panais
champignons

WHY DO WE **GAIN WEIGHT?**

Our era is one of paradoxes! On one hand the life expectancy of humans continues to increase and on the other their health continues to deteriorate. There are two reasons for this.

The first is genetic. Based on Darwin's law, in the past only the strongest individuals survived and had physically robust descendants. Nowadays, thanks to progress in modern medicine, everyone survives. Natural selection no longer occurs, the human species has become weaker and weaker and bodies are much less resistant and thus more vulnerable.

The second reason for the poor health of humans at present, is because the nutritional quality of our diet has considerably declined over the last fifty years, due to its industrialization. Moreover, we have to admit that the same period has been dominated by a slow slide in our eating habits, resulting in our unwitting change in the nature of what we eat.

The remarkable increase in metabolic diseases (obesity, diabetes and cardiovascular disease) over the last decades just confirms this.

Worldwide obesity epidemic

In June 1997, WHO (World Health Organization) finally decided to sound the alarm by reporting an increase of obesity in the world, which had become a real epidemic. The entire world is now involved. Industrial countries (in particular in the United States), but also all developing nations.

In 1910, the proportion of obese people was basically the same everywhere. It was 3% for the United States and Germany and 2% for the other European nations, including France, which was more or less as it had been for centuries. Twenty-five years later, in 1935, the proportion of obese people had almost doubled everywhere, except in the United States where it had tripled. After World War II, not only had the upward trend been confirmed, but it had worsened in an alarming manner in the United States where the percentage of obese people was already 16%.

WORLDWIDE OBESITY IN 1997 (WHO)

- United States: 33%
- Germany: 22%
- India: 20%
- United Kingdom: 16%
- Spain: 9%
- France: 8.5%

WHO's 1997 warning doesn't seem to have changed things much. And ten years later, in 2007, the situation is even worse. The United States now reports 36% obese in their population and France is, according to the last official ObEpi (epidemiological obesity) survey published in 2009, at 12.5%, which means an increase of 47% in ten years for the country!

OBESITY IN YOUNG PEOPLE:

Obesity is even more preoccupying for younger generations. Childhood obesity has risen in the last ten years by 22% in France, 40% in Great Britain and 60% in the United States, but also, which is even more surprising, by 53% in Japan, 75% in Singapore and 250% in China.

How did this happen? And what are health-care officials in the various countries doing to stem this progression?

The official nutritional message for 50 years

There has been an official nutritional message for half a century. This message, which started out in the United States in the 1930's before being adopted everywhere, is based

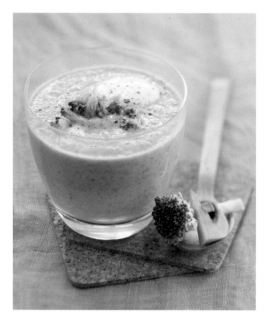

on a hypothesis which consists of thinking that if people are heavier it is for two reasons:

• they eat too much (in calories) and particularly too much fat;

• they don't move enough. People have actually become too sedentary and do not exercise enough to use the calories they consume.
The result is an imbalance between inputs (of energy) and outputs.

Starting from this hypothesis, two recommendations were made:

• eat less (in calories) to prevent gaining weight;

• go on a diet to lose weight.
In both cases, it was also recommended to move more by exercising.

And this is what they did, not just in the United States - where one third of the population diets from January 1st to December 31st -, but also in all other countries, mainly European, where they intend limiting the increase of the generally overweight in the population and even more obesity.

Yet after more than half a century of official, widespread practice of this energy balance, the prevalence of obesity has multiplied by four. So one can legitimately question its validity.

Examination of the official nutritional hypothesis

For more than twenty years, numerous epidemiological studies have made it possible to understand the possible effectiveness of official nutritional recommendations.

And here, we see numerous paradoxes.

1 – The average daily energy consumption in industrialized countries has decreased 30 to 35% in half a century.

Paradoxically, the prevalence of obesity has increased more than 300% during the same period. In France, the decrease in energy intake has been 36% since 1960 and 50% since 1935.

2 – The obese do not eat more than their normal weight counterparts.

If anything it is the opposite. The statistics of Professor Creff also show that more than 51% of the obese eat less and even far less than the average.

3 – The obese do not use less energy.

Unlike what has long been believed, the obese do not use less energy. The opposite is true, the obese use more energy than a comparable person (height, age), due to their excess weight.

4 – Numerous obese people have a significant physical consumption.

In western countries, agricultural workers, craftsmen and workers are heavier than those who work in offices. In Russia, 56% of women over age 30 are obese, despite the fact that their energy intake is low (around 1,500 Kcal) and most of them do physical work.

5 – Poor people are more likely to be overweight and obese, despite the fact that they do not eat more than the average.

This is the case in all western countries, and particularly the United States. On the contrary, the richer people are, the thinner they are.

6 – Numerous developing countries have an alarming obesity level (and diabetes).

This is the case of India, where more than 20% of the population is obese, despite the fact that Indians – becoming more and more numerous – do not eat more than before.

IN CONCLUSION

There is no correlation between the quantity of calories eaten on average per day by a given population and the level of corpulence of the same population. In other words the energy factor is not determinant in gaining weight.

The nutritional characteristic of a food

Thus the nutritional hypothesis of energy balance between calorie intake on one hand and consumption on the other seems to be totally incorrect. The biggest error was to consider that all of the calories calculated "in the plate" had the same value and are automatically available in the body. Yet, in light of current knowledge on the digestive physiology of foods and the nature of metabolic mechanisms which occur, it is now easy to understand how things really work. Thus, it was then shown that what is important in a food is not its QUANTITY (measured in calories) but its QUALITY, i.e. its nutritional characteristic.

The nutritional characteristic of a food is determined by three criteria:

• its **nutritional content**, both macronutrients (carbohydrates, fats and proteins) and micronutrients (vitamins, minerals, trace elements, fiber and essential fatty acids);

• its **intestinal absorption** rate which measures the nutritional bioavailability of a food;

• its **metabolic potential** which measures the range of carbohydrate and insulin response, as well as the incidence on thermogenesis (energy expenditure caused by digestion).

200 Kcal of potatoes are not 200 Kcal of lentils

Let's take two plates.

In the first we'll put 220 g of potatoes, i.e. 200 Kcal.

In the second we'll put 180 g of lentils (cooked), i.e. 200 Kcal.

For a traditional nutritionist, these two food portions are nutritionally identical, even if the weight of the lentils is slightly lower. This is because the potatoes and the lentils are two carbohydrates, and moreover complex carbohydrates. Consequently the calorie content (carbohydrate) is the same (200 Kcal), whether one eats one or the other is the same for the traditional nutritionist, since the two portions for him are interchangeable.

The physiological reality is completely different. Let's see why:

Consumption of 200 Kcal of potatoes

Taking into account the nature of the potato starch (high proportion of amylopectin, low proportion of amylose), digestion of a potato by the digestive enzymes (hydrolization) is around 80%.

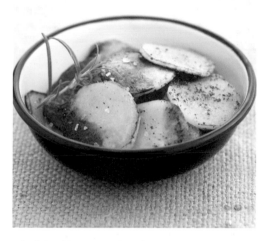

This means that 80% of the 200 Kcal of starch are transformed into glucose, which crosses the intestinal wall to enter the blood.

As we know, glycemia (fasting) is around 1 g of glucose (sugar) per liter of blood. Yet, as soon as a carbohydrate is consumed, after it is transformed into glucose it enters the blood. When the glycemic peak is reached, it starts a proportional insulin secretion, used to lower the glycemia. Glucose is then stored in the liver and muscle tissues (glycogen), where it can be later used as fuel.

Thus, in the case of the potato, the digestion of 200 Kcal of starch results in a significant increase in glycemia followed by a significant secretion of insulin. Around 80% of starch is transformed into glucose, so we can consider that 160 Kcal are available (in terms of energy) in the body in comparison to the 200 Kcal

which had been on the plate.

Consumption of 200 Kcal of lentils

Taking into account the nature of the lentil starch (low proportion of amylopectin, high proportion of amylose), digestion of lentils by the digestive enzymes (hydrolization) is only around 20 %.

This means that only 20 % of the 200 Kcal of starch are transformed into glucose, which crosses the intestinal wall to enter the blood.

Thus only a very low increase in glycemia is started followed by a very low, or even zero, insulin secretion.

Around only 20 % of starch is transformed into glucose, so we can consider that only 40 Kcal

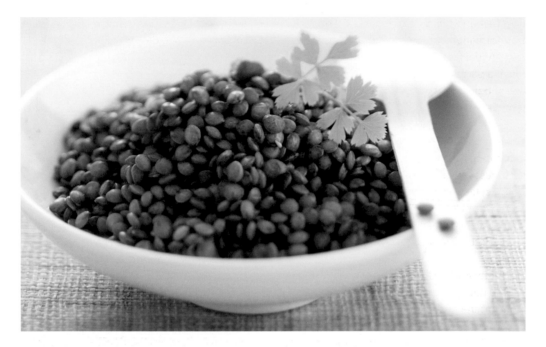

are available (in terms of energy) in the body in comparison to the 200 Kcal which had been on the plate.

The first observation which is clear is that by consuming 200 Kcal of lentils, the energy actually available to the body is four times less than what we obtain by eating a portion of potatoes with the same number of calories. In other words the food calories calculated in the plate have nothing to do with those which are actually available in the body after digestion. For a comparable food, this may range from single to quadruple.

Two carbohydrates are not interchangeable

The metabolic responses which follow eating of two portions of potatoes and lentils with the same number of calories are completely different, very high for the potatoes and very low for the lentils.

Furthermore each of these metabolic responses in turn starts other metabolic consequents, which may result in gaining weight or inversely losing weight.

In the case of the potato, taking into account the significant glycemia and the strong insulin response, it is likely that the excess of glucose (compared to the glycogen needs) causes a transformation into fat and storage, or weight gain. And if fats were eaten during the same meal, a part of these fatty acids has a strong risk of being transformed into stored fat due to hyperinsulinism, starting additional weight gain.

In the case of lentils, the low glycemia (four times less than that of potatoes) is without doubt sufficient for satisfying glycogen needs. Moreover, given the low insulin response, neither the glucose (because there is no excess) nor the accompanying fats will be stored as fat.

Thus fatty acids will be used normally for the energy needs of the body. And if they are significant the body also manages by increasing to consume its PPEE (postprandial energy expenditure). But in the hypothesis where fatty acids would be insufficient, the body would automatically start another metabolic process (lypolysis) consisting of drawing its energy from the stored fats, starting a weight loss.

Moreover, eating potatoes results in hyperglycemia and hyperinsulinism, the level of fullness is not satisfactory and there is a **risk of reactionary hypoglycemia** after around two hours, where the main symptoms are fatigue (after-meal fatigue) and hunger. This causes a temptation to snack.

On the contrary, this risk does not exist with lentils, where their consumption contributes to an excellent sensation of fullness, which lasts until the next meal. There is no risk of reactionary hypoglycemia, due to the low secretion of insulin.

In conclusion, we can say that unlike what nutritionalists have long believed, two carbohydrates are not interchangeable. The more resistant a starch is, the less the absorption of glucose (thus its low bioavailability) and paradoxically, the higher the level of fullness. We could also add that the risk of gaining weight is lower, no matter what fats are consumed at the same time. This is because it is now important to choose carbohydrates based on a new criterion: the glycemic index.

"SLOW SUGARS" AND "FAST SUGARS": AN INCORRECT IDEA!

For a long time nutritionists have classified carbohydrates in two categories: simple carbohydrates (or "fast absorbing sugars", fast sugars) and complex carbohydrates (or "slow absorbing sugars", slow sugars).
Yet, more than fifteen years ago it was demonstrated that this classification is totally wrong! Experiments showed that all carbohydrates, whether simple or complex, are absorbed within the same timeframe (around half an hour) and that the mistake they made was to mix up the food digestion speed with the absorption speed.

The glycemic index (GI)

The classification of carbohydrates is thus now done based on their hyperglycemizing power which corresponds, as we saw earlier, to the absorption rate of their sugars, whether they are single/double or complex. This new classification starts with the idea of glycemic index.

The glycemic index of a carbohydrate measures its bioavailability in a scale of values composed by taking pure glucose (100% bioavailable) to which a value of 100 is given.

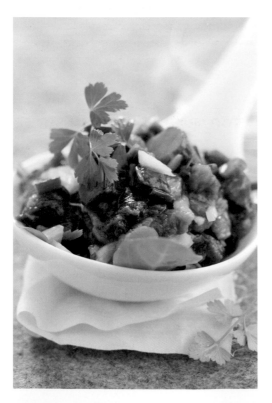

All carbohydrates are then measured based on their hyperglycemizing power compared to that of glucose. Consequently, in the glycemic index range, French fries are at 95, whereas lentils only have an index of 30.

If one carefully observes the glycemic index table, one will note that all of the carbohydrates with a high GI (on page 22) are refined foods (flour, sugar, rice, etc.), industrially processed foods (corn flakes, puffed rice, modified starches, energy bars, etc.) or "new" foods, i.e. which have only been regularly eaten for less than two centuries, such as potatoes, white flours or even sugar.

Yet, one must admit that all of these foods are precisely those which are currently most eaten in most western countries, and which, progressively, due to globalization, are invading the eating habits of other countries.

Conversely, if one observes page 23, i.e. the one for low glycemic index, one sees that the foods listed there mostly correspond to products which are barely no longer eaten nowadays (whole wheat bread, complete grains, unrefined flours, brown rice, etc.), food which are eaten on an increasingly rare basis (lentils, dry beans, split peas, chick peas, etc.) or even less (fruit, green vegetables, etc.). Yet they are all foods that were eaten much more in the past, even just fifty years ago.

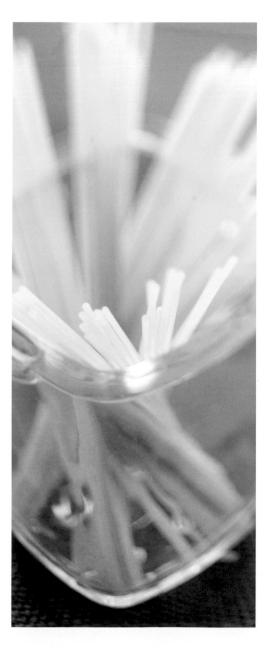

Hyperinsulinism

A constantly hyperglycemizing diet (based on the consumption of high GI carbohydrates), which corresponds to a modern diet, leads to hyperinsulinism, i.e. an excessive secretion of insulin, one of the key hormones of metabolism.

Yet, it has been shown that hyperinsulinism is not only responsible for gaining weight (in particular from preferential storage of fats consumed at the same time) but it is also a factor in the development of diabetes and a certain number of cardiovascular diseases (cholesterol, high blood pressure, triglycerides, etc.).

TOO MUCH GLUCOSE CAUSES WEIGHT GAIN

Moreover, we have to be aware that due to their sedentary nature, modern individuals only need a very small amount if glucose. Yet, by eating carbohydrates with a high GI, they are paradoxically eating more than their ancestors did of low GI carbohydrates, even if their needs are half.
This excessive glucose is then automatically transformed into fat, which means gaining weight.

Carbohydrates with high glycemic index (GI ≥ 55)

Maltose (beer)	110	Sugary refined grains	70
Glucose	100	Chocolate bars	70
Baked potatoes	95	Boiled, peeled potatoes	70
French fries	95	Carbonated soft drinks	70
Rice flour	95	Cookies	70
Modified starches	95	Modern corn	70
Mashed potato	90	White rice	70
Chips	90	Pasta, ravioli	70
Honey	85	Raisins	65
White hamburger buns	85	Brown bread	65
Cooked carrots	85	Boiled, unpeeled potatoes	65
Corn flakes, pop corn	85	Beet	65
Instant/parboiled rice	85	Jam (with sugar added)	65
Rice cake	85	Cream of wheat	60
Puffed rice (Rice crispies)	85	Long grain white/brown rice	60
Cooked fava beans	80	Banana	60
Pumpkin	75	Melon	60
Watermelon	75	Well-cooked white spaghetti	55
Sugar (saccharose)	70	Shortbread	55
White bread (baguettes)	70		

Carbohydrates with low glycemic index (GI ≤ 50)

Brown rice	50	Lettuce	30
Long grain basmati rice	50	Dried white beans	30
Sweet potato	50	Lentils (brown or yellow)	30
Whole grain pasta	50	Chick peas	30
Al dente spaghetti	45	Other fresh fruit (apples, pears, oranges,	30
Fresh peas	40	apricots, etc.)	30
Compete grains without sugar	40	Green beans	30
Oatmeal	40	Soy noodles	30
Kidney beans	40	Stewed fruit (without sugar)	22
Fresh fruit juice (no added sugar)	40	Green lentils	22
Pumpernickel bread	40	Flageolet beans	22
Whole grain rye bread	40	Split pea	22
100% whole-wheat bread	40	Dark chocolate (> 70 % cacao)	22
Alginate ice	40	Fructose	20
Al dente whole wheat pasta	40	Soy	15
Dried fig, dried apricot	35	Cashew	15
Indian corn	35	Fresh apricots	15
Wild rice	35	Green vegetables, salad, tomato	< 15
Quinoa	35	Eggplant, zucchini, garlic, onion, etc.	< 15
Raw carrot	30	You can find the glycemic index of many other foods on the website **www.montignac.com**	

THE METHOD'S **DIETARY PRINCIPLES**

First of all the Montignac method is a different way of eating. Unlike what some detractors would like you to believe, it cannot be considered as a diet, since it does not involve limiting quantity. It simply leads to refocusing eating habits: **you don't eat less, you just eat better!**

It mainly consists of selecting foods based on their nutritional characteristics and their metabolic potential.

Selecting foods

Carbohydrates
These will mostly be selected from those whose GI is low in order to prevent an excessive increase of glycemia, which causes a critical insulin response that starts the weight gain mechanism. But experience has shown that eating carbohydrates with a GI lower than or equal to 35 (see the table on pg. 23) leads to weight loss and decrease of risk factors for diabetes and cardiovascular diseases. Permanent results are later obtained by maintaining an average glycemia outcome during the meal.

Fats
Fats will be primarily chosen from monounsaturated (olive oil, goose and duck fat) and animal polyunsaturated (omega-3 fish oil) fatty acids. These acids improve weight loss and contribute to decreasing cardiovascular risk factors unlike saturated fats (butter, margarine, meat fat, lard, etc.)

Proteins:
These will be chosen based on their origin (animal or vegetable) and their neutrality compared to insulin response. Moreover they will be eaten in a sufficient quantity (around 30% of total energy intake). Proteins permit a better sensation of fullness and help increase basic energy consumption.

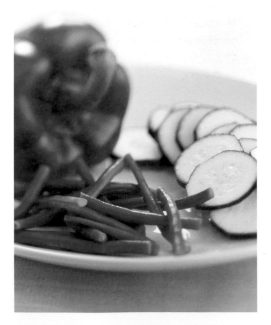

SCIENTIFICALLY PROVEN EFFECTIVENESS

The Montignac method's legitimacy stems from the combined wisdom of numerous scientific studies published in the last twenty years, but also from the testimonies of ten of thousands of people, including doctors who prescribe it in France and another forty countries.

It is part of a current of international scientific thought where some great epidemiologists are leaders, for example Professor Walter Willett of Harvard Medical School.

The Montignac method has shown its proof in terms of effectiveness (short and long term) and beneficial secondary effects, as shown in specific studies (Canadian study by Professor Dumesnil published in November 2001 in the British Journal of Nutrition).

It is currently the only credible solution to the low calorie diet, that of despair and failure that has been proposed to us to date and whose nutritional recommendations are, according to Professor Willett, largely responsible for the explosion of obesity in the world.

The method's two phases

Phase I: weight loss phase
This period varies according to how much weight is to be lost. In addition to wisely selecting fats and proteins, it primarily involves only eating (in terms of carbohydrates) those foods whose glycemic index (GI) is lower than or equal to 35. The goal is to have the lowest insulin response at the end of each meal. This not only removes any chance of storage (lipogenesis) but just the reverse; it activates the process of removing fat from stores (lipolysis), so that it is burned when energy use (thermogenesis) increases.

Phase II: stabilization and prevention phase
Carbohydrates will still be selected according to their GI but the selection will be broader than in phase I.

The choices can even be refined by using a new concept, that of a meal's glycemic load (synthesis between GI and the food's pure carbohydrate content) and above all the meal's **glycemic outcome** (GO). This means that all carbohydrates can be eaten under some conditions, even those with high GI.

THE GLYCEMIC OUTCOME (GO)

The Go is the average rise in glyce-mia obtained at the end of a complex meal, due to the interaction of the various foods which compose it.

This new concept acts as a guide in phase II. So thanks to this concept it is possible to eat a high GI carbohydrate during a meal, by neutralizing a signifi-cant part of its effects on glycemia, as long as mainly very low GI carbohydra-tes are first eaten to create a compen-sation phenomenon.

You can also consider that in phase II, all foods, with no exception, can be eaten.

Meal structure

The basic principle consists of making three meals per day:
• a breakfast;
• a lunch;
• a dinner;
There are two types of meals: fat-protein meals and carbohydrate-protein meals.

Fat-protein meal (or lipidic)

This contains proteins and fats (meats, eggs, cheeses, etc.), but also carbohydrates with a glycemic index which must be lower than or equal to 35.

Carbohydrate-protein meal (or glucidic)

This is basically composed of carbohydrates whose glycemic index is between 35 and 50 (for example spaghetti). In addition to the proteins already present in the carbohydrates,

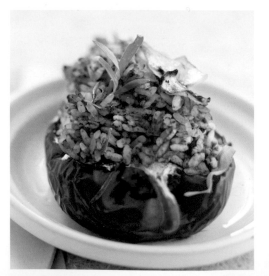

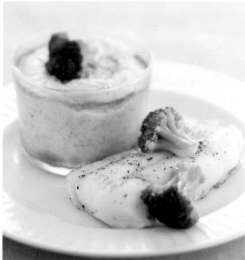

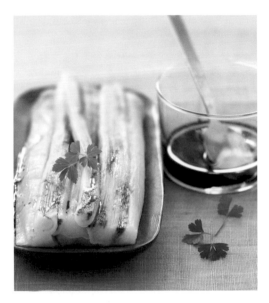

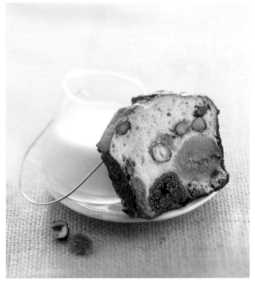

you can also add others, as long as they do not contain saturated fats (chicken or turkey ham, dried beef, etc.). The only fats allowed in a carbohydrate meal are omega-3 oils (raw, poached or steamed fish) and a half portion of monounsaturated fats (olive oil drizzled on the spaghetti).

The eating balance is made (unless otherwise indicated/stated) over the day:

• Breakfast is **carbohydrate-protein** (see pg. 34).

• Lunch is the main meal and is **fat-protein** and includes:
- an appetizer (raw vegetables);
- a main dish composed of proteins and fats (meats, poultry, fish and eggs) and a carbohydrate with GI equal to or less than 35 (green vegetables, lentils, green beans, peas, etc.);

- a dessert composed of fruit, cheese or a preparation (cake, desserts, etc.) with a GI equal to or less than 35.

• Dinner in principle is lighter and, three times out of five, is **carbohydrate-protein**, it includes:
- an appetizer (optional), for example vegetable soup;
- a carbohydrate dish (spaghetti, lentils, rice, etc.);
- a dessert (optional): fruit and fat-free yogurt.

But it is completely possible to invert the meal types during the day, particularly for work reasons, by making dinner the main meal, then lunch will become lighter.

THE METHOD'S **CULINARY PRINCIPLES**

All of the recipes in this book comply with the Montignac method. They are all phase I recipes, i.e. those that can be used immediately in the weight loss phase.

Thus, none of them contain bad carbohydrates (with a high GI). In contrast, the ingredients which are proposed – and the side dishes – have a low or even very low glycemic index (less than or equal to 35).

Moreover, with a few exceptions, all of the recipes in this book are inspired on Mediterranean and in particular Provencal cuisine. I really like the cuisine of the sun. This is a weakness I have always had, but I was able to discover all of the subtleties and appreciate the incomparable fragrances over many years, since I had the chance to live in southeast France and spend my vacations on Corsica. It is also a simple cuisine, easy and fast to make, where the flavors are popular throughout the world, regardless of cultural background. Lastly, it is a healthy cuisine, i.e. where all the ingredients are to a large extent beneficial for health, particularly for preventing metabolic diseases (obesity, diabetes and cardiovascular disease).

The 3 bad students of traditional cuisine

As you'll quickly realize, three of the main ingredients of traditional cuisine are completely absent in these recipes, including and above all in desserts: white flour, sugar and butter.

Flour and sugar
These are naturally avoided because they are carbohydrates with a very high glycemic index.

Butter
It is excluded because it is a bad fat (saturated fatty acids), especially when it is cooked. Nevertheless, all or almost all cookbooks propose butter as a cooking fat. Even in the great classics of Provencal cuisine, butter is often indicated in a large number of recipes. Butter was once a rare, expensive product, thus noble. Cuisine with butter at that time was the privilege of the wealthy (aristocrats and upper middle classes) and was consequently largely developed by the cooks who served them. France's gastronomy tradition, inherited from that epoch, is thus mainly based on cuisine with butter.
If butter is acceptable in a nutritional program (around 10 to 20 g per day) when it is eaten raw or slightly melted, this is absolutely not true when it is cooked.
Butter is basically composed of saturated fats, composed of "short chain" fatty acids which have the advantage of being quickly

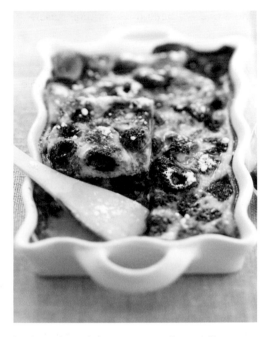

or 180° C or even higher, which is a temperature completely unacceptable for butter.

It is not the same thing for the other fats which we wholeheartedly recommend: olive oil and goose or duck fat.

Olive oil

Mentioned constantly in the Bible, olive oil was an essential food in ancient civilizations. Our ancestors did not just use it for eating and lighting, but also for treatment. But for many centuries, it remained the poor fat of mainly Mediterranean countries. By the middle of the 20th century, it had practically fallen out of use and been replaced by "modern" fats: sunflower oil, corn oil and margarine.

After having then spent a few centuries rejected by western cuisine, olive oil has made a strong comeback in recent decades in our culinary practices. It has also slowly refound its illustrious past thanks to its aura of healthiness, primarily rediscovered in light of scientific studies on the famous Mediterranean diet, but also thanks to the talent of great chefs, such as Alain Ducasse.

The critical temperature of olive oil (when it starts to smoke) is much higher than for other types of oil. Thus, based on its acidity content, it can be heated to 230°C, while peanut oil cannot exceed 200°C, sunflower

broken down by enzymes in the small intestine. This is why chilled butter is fairly easy to digest. But when it reaches a temperature of 100°C, these famous short chain fatty acids are progressively destroyed. This is why cooked butter is indigestible, since it cannot be broken down normally by the enzymes in the small intestine.

It also constitutes an additional health risk factor. In addition to its negative impact on cholesterol and the risk of clogging arteries, cooked butter (from 100°C) produces acrolein, recognized as a carcinogen.
Yet, when a knob of butter is put in a skillet or a pan on a burner, to make a traditional recipe, the temperature quickly rises to 160

oil 170°C and butter only 110°C.
Olive oil is thus intentionally omnipresent in this recipe book where it is used both hot and cold.

Goose (or duck) fat

Some may be surprised that it is possible to sing the praises of such a fat, even though nutritionalists have long told us that good fats are vegetable and bad ones are animal. Yet, it has long been scientifically proven that this dichotomy is totally false.

Certain vegetable fats, such as palm oil, are harmful because they are highly saturated, while certain animal fats are highly beneficial, this is the case of goose and duck fat. These fats basically have the same chemical structure as olive oil. They are essentially composed of oleic acid, a monounsaturated fatty acid.

Goose fat thus has two big advantages. It has the same properties of olive oil (very high melting point, cardiovascular prevention factor, etc.) and it gives dishes exceptional flavors which results in very tasty plates.

Soy cream

In many of the recipes soy cream is proposed in place of liquid crème fraîche. The product can be used to make a creamy sauce avoiding the saturated fat in crème fraîche. It goes well with vegetables and fish. If used with meats, it is best to enhance the flavor with goose fat.

The only problem with soy cream is that it turns quickly making lumps if it is cooked over a high flame or for too long. So it does not do well if simmered. Thus it is better to add it at the end of cooking or to a sauce cooked in a double-boiler. A tip: First deglaze the cooking surface with a little water then add the cream heating very slightly (over a low flame or in a double-boiler) without cooking.

Nutritional gastronomy

This recipe book, like the earlier ones, is largely inspired on the "nutritional gastronomy" concept which I developed more than twenty years ago.

Up to then, the dietary landscape was divided into two groups where each representative considered the frontier with an exacerbated Manicheism. On one hand there was the Rabelaisian world of the "huge spread", that of unending banquets, plates overflowing with fatty, tasty victuals. This was the time of "bon vivants" where a love of life and existential well-being was measured by their ruddy faces and the width of their waists. It was the privileged world of the gastronomy of abundance, gourmets and food lovers who without concern and with Epicureanism dug their graves with their forks.

And then, on the other hand, there was (and still is) the puritan and sadomasochistic world of traditional dieting, that of forbidden items, symbolic frugal portions and above all low-calories, odorless, bland and tasteless foods, protein powder appetite suppressants and meal replacements.

This was (and still is) the world for those who think eating is almost a sin. It is a world of sad people, killjoys and spoilsports, killjoys of eating when hungry, those who try to give you a guilty conscience and those who with one glance can kill your appetite.

And in other words, it is the world which, under the pretext of lengthening your life, forbids you from even enjoying living.

"Nutritional gastronomy" is an attempt to reconcile these two enemies. It is a middle ground between food debauchery and asceticism. It starts with the idea that eating, in addition to being a physiological necessity, should be a pleasure, that it is an action that should be part of the quality of life. It denounces any restrictive approach leading to deprivation of nourishment and severely condemns any practice consisting of suppressing the appetite and trying to meet the body's needs with artifices such as meal replacements.

GOOD FOOD SENSE

"Nutritional gastronomy" is "eating well", "eating pleasure" and "eating healthy". It is a return to a certain good food sense. It is "eating intelligently" which consists of keeping the best of the gastronomical tradition but based on current nutritional scientific knowledge that challenges the accepted ideas of a totally outdated diet. This is the combination of "eating well" and "eating healthy".

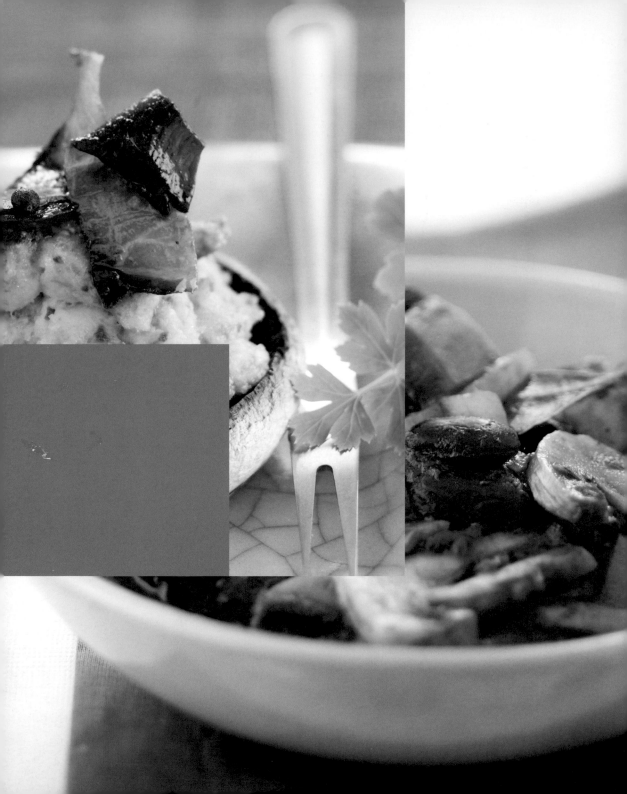

EVERYDAY
MENUS

You will find 8 weeks of Montignac menus below composed of all of the recipes in this book. All of these menus comply with the principles of the Montignac method. They are essentially a guideline and actually show how to divide food choices over the day and week to achieve a balanced diet (30% proteins, 30% fats and 40% carbohydrates), including taking into account the intake from breakfast which is mainly carbohydrates.

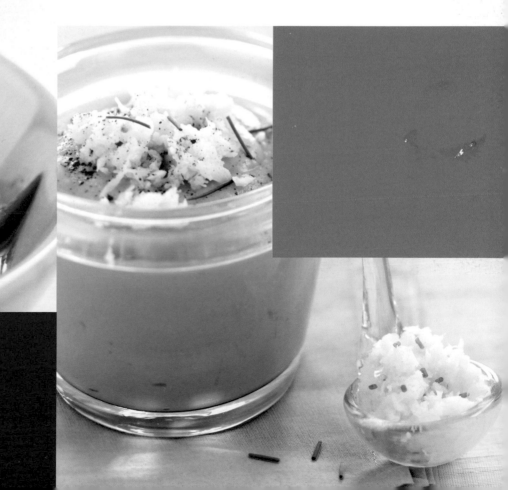

TWO MONTHS OF **MONTIGNAC MENUS**

Breakfast

The menus below only give guidelines for organizing the main meals: lunch and dinner. The morning meal was intentionally left out, since aside from a few changes is it basically always the same.

Nevertheless, it is important that it be organized according to the principles of the Montignac method[1].

It is basically carbohydrate-protein in nature. Thus it includes:

Carbohydrates with a low glycemic index:
• fruits;
• whole-wheat bread[2], rye crackers with 24% fiber and Pumpernickel;
• unrefined cereals without sugar;
• jam without sugar3.

Proteins:
• fat-free yogurt;
• fat-free cheese;
• chicken or turkey ham;
• smoked or marinated salmon.

A drink
Decaffeinated coffee, Arabican coffee, cocoa, chicory, skimed milk; soy and almond milk; tea and tisanes and fresh fruit juice with the pulp (avoid industrial juices from concentrate and sweetened) are recommended.

• Sugar and all saturated fats (particularly butter) are to be absolutely avoided.

Lunch

This is the most important meal. It is according to Montignac terminology "**fat-protein**", which means that it contains fats (generally good fats) and proteins from different sources (meats, fish, eggs, cheese, etc.) and carbohydrates (vegetables, pulses, grains and cereals whose glycemic index is less than or equal to 35).

Lunch is normally composed of three dishes:

• An appetizer: in almost all cases this is a vegetable, especially raw.

• An entree: composed of a meat, fish or egg dish, served with a cooked vegetable.

• A dessert: entails four different formulas to choose from:
- a cheese served with a salad;
- fruit or a fruit dish;
- a yogurt;
- a "Montignac" dessert, i.e. without flour, saturated fats (butter) and without sugar (possibly replaced by fructose).

Dinner

The evening meal in turn is lighter, meaning less plentiful and it has a higher carbohydrate content. Three dinners per week are **carbo-hydrate-protein** (CP), they do not contain any fat, except for fish oil or a symbolic quantity of olive oil.
Sunday always involves a more festive and plentiful meal than the other days of the week, this in keeping with the family tradition.

Dinner, with a more significant carbohydrate composition, only includes two dishes: an entree and a dessert, since by principle, and with the occasional exception, the evening meal should be lighter.

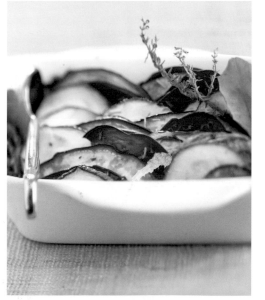

GOOD TO KNOW

• These menus are a guideline, this means that not only can the days be inverted, but it is also always possible to switch lunch with dinner.

• Lunch or dinner can be substituted with a Montignac snack, in particular:
- A sandwich on whole-wheat bread[4] with a very low glycemic index composed on raw vegetables and/or smoked salmon or fat-free proteins like chicken or turkey ham, or hardboiled egg white.
- Fresh or dried fruit which can be eaten with hazelnuts, walnuts and in particular almonds.

1. For additional information see books by Michel Montignac: *Eat yourself slim*, Alpen Editions, 2010. *Glycemic Index Diet*, Alpen Editions, 2010. *The Montignac Diet Cookbook*, Alpen Editions, 2010.
2. See the website www.montignac-shop.com to get whole wheat bread.
3. See the website www.montignac-shop.com to get jam without sugar.
4. Only the real Montignac integral bread is acceptable in this case as long as it is the only whole-wheat bread to have the lowest GI in the world (34). You may get this exceptional bread through the website www.montignac-shop.com

WEEK 1

	Salmon filet with olive cream (pg.132)	Pork chops with green lentils (pg. 180)	Poellée de st jacques (scallops) aux échalottes (pg. 120)
	MONDAY	**TUESDAY**	**WEDNESDAY**
Breakfast	See pg. 34	See pg. 34	See pg. 34
Lunch	• Tomatoes with mozzarella • Salmon filet with olive cream (pg. 132) • Spinach • Cheese	• Cucumber with soy cream. • Pork chops with green lentils (pg. 180) • Berries	• Endive salad with walnuts • Poêlée de Saint-Jacques aux écha-lotes (pg. 120) • Peas • 2 or 3 squares of chocolate with more than 70% cocoa
Dinner	• Spaghetti with basil tomato sauce (pg. 220) • Yogurt CP	• Chicken breast with parmesan (pg. 160) • Green salad • Custard with fructose	• Vegetarian stuffed tomatoes (pg. 204) • Basmati rice • Compote CP

CP: carbohydrate-protein meal

Cream of avocado soup with crab (pg. 60)	Chicken breast with curry (pg. 158)	Quinoa tabouli (pg. 72)	Nectarine cake with almonds (pg. 252)
THURSDAY	**FRIDAY**	**SATURDAY**	**SUNDAY**
See pg. 34	See pg. 34	See pg. 34	See pg. 34
• Cream of avocado soup with crab (pg. 60) • Cod with broccoli (pg. 144) • Fromage blanc drained	• Salade d'épinards à la sévillane (pg. 71) • Chicken breast with curry (pg. 158) • Yogurt	• Quinoa tabouli (pg. 72) • Tuna filet with tomato (pg. 138) • Salad • Cheese	• Salade landaise (pg. 70) • Rack of lamb with champignons (pg. 188) • Green salad • Cheese • Nectarine cake with almonds (pg. 252)
• Omelet with champignons • Green salad • Cheese	• Bell peppers stuffed with ewe cheese (pg. 86) • Baked apple CP	• Cured ham • Tian à la provençale (pg. 214) • Three fruit cake (pg. 244)	• Green lentil terrine (pg. 92) • Soft-boiled egg • Yogurt

CP: carbohydrate-protein meal

WEEK 2

Snow peas
with bacon
(pg. 216)

Tuna filet
with ginger
(pg. 128)

Vegetarian chili
(pg. 202)

	MONDAY	TUESDAY	WEDNESDAY
Breakfast	See pg. 34	See pg. 34	See pg. 34
Lunch	• Endive salad with walnuts • Pork chop • Snow peas with bacon (pg. 216) • Custard with fructose	• Grated carrots dressed with lemon juice • Tuna filet with ginger (pg. 128) • Fresh cheese	• Radishes • Foies de volaille à la provençale (pg. 162) • Yogurt
Dinner	• Spaghetti with basil tomato sauce (pg. 220) • Baked apple CP	• Quinoa tabouli (pg. 72) • Smoked salmon • Yogurt	• Vegetarian chili (pg. 202) • Compote CP

CP: carbohydrate-protein meal

Omelet with eggplants (pg. 190)	Chilled cucumber soup with green apples (pg. 68)	Prune mousse (pg. 236)	Foie gras terrine (pg. 94)
THURSDAY	**FRIDAY**	**SATURDAY**	**SUNDAY**
See pg. 34	See pg. 34	See pg. 34	See pg. 34
• Cucumber salad Beef with paprika (pg. 186) • Broccoli • Plain strawberries	• Chilled broccoli soup (pg. 66) • Skewers of two fish (pg. 151) • Green beans • Soy milk yogurt	• Gratin de courgette à la grecque (pg. 88) • Red mullet with anchoïade (pg. 130) • Prune mousse (pg. 236)	• Foie gras terrine (pg. 94) • Saint-Jacques aux champignons (pg. 124) • Clafoutis aux framboises (pg. 246)
• Omelet with eggplant (pg. 190) • Green salad • Cheese	• Chilled cucumber soup with green apples (pg. 68) • Sliced turkey • Lentils • Poached pear CP	• Leek soup • Fried egg • Green salad • Berries	• Stuffed champignons (pg. 170) • Salad • Cheese

CP: carbohydrate-protein meal

WEEK 3

Spaghetti with basil tomato sauce (pg. 220)

plain raspberry

Avocado soup (pg. 64)

	MONDAY	TUESDAY	WEDNESDAY
Breakfast	See pg. 34	See pg. 34	See pg. 34
Lunch	• Red cabbage salad • Veal liver seasoned with parsley • Green beans • Fruit	• Greek salad (tomatoes + feta) • Slice of lamb • Flageolet beans • Yogurt	• Avocado soup (pg. 64) • Tuna with tomato and olives (pg. 142) • Broccoli • Salad • Cheese
Dinner	• Spaghetti with basil tomato sauce (pg. 220) • Yogurt CP	• Steamed artichoke • Cheese omelet • Plain raspberries	• Green lentils • Steamed salmon • Compote CP

CP: carbohydrate-protein meal

Chicken livers sautéed in ginger (pg. 156)	Bell peppers stuffed with basmati rice (pg. 198)	Chicken with pastis and fennel (pg. 164)	Bitter chocolate fondant (pg. 228)
THURSDAY	**FRIDAY**	**SATURDAY**	**SUNDAY**
See pg. 34	See pg. 34	See pg. 34	See pg. 34
• Champignons with vinaigrette • Chicken livers sautéed in ginger (pg. 156) • Celery puree • Compote	• White leek salad with vinaigrette (pg. 78) • Monkfish with spinach (pg. 150) • Custard with fructose	• Clafoutis d'oignons (pg. 104) • Chicken with pastis and fennel (pg. 164) • Goat cheese cake (pg. 242)	• Duck breast tartare (pg. 106) • Sea bass with fennel (pg. 148) • Broccoli • Bitter chocolate fondant (pg. 228)
• Grated carrots dressed with lemon juice • Poached trout • Broccoli • Yogurt	• Bell peppers stuffed with basmati rice (pg. 198) • Prunes CP	• Shrimp gratin (pg. 118) • Green salad • Cheese	• Stuffed eggplants à la provençale (pg. 196) • Compote à l'ancienne (pg. 235)

CP: carbohydrate-protein meal

WEEK 4

	Cod with broccoli (pg. 144)	Leek quiche (pg. 102)	Tuna filet with tomato (pg. 138)
	MONDAY	**TUESDAY**	**WEDNESDAY**
Breakfast	See pg. 34	See pg. 34	See pg. 34
Lunch	• Avocado dressed with vinaigrette • Cod with broccoli (pg. 144) • Green salad • Raspberries	• Céleri rémoulade (celeriac, fat-free yogurt and mustard) • Omelet andalouse (pg. 194) • Green salad • Cheese	• Heart of palm • Tuna filet with tomato (pg. 138) • Broccoli • Yogurt
Dinner	• Spaghetti with basil tomato sauce (pg. 220) • Apple compote CP	• Avocado dressed with vinaigrette • Leek quiche (pg. 102) • Peach	• Omelet made with egg whites, tomato and turkey ham • Bean sprouts • Lemon juice CP

CP: carbohydrate-protein meal

Hanger steak on grated shallots (pg. 184)	White leek salad with vinaigrette (pg. 78)	croque-aubergine (pg. 168)	Clafoutis aux framboises (pg. 246)
THURSDAY	**FRIDAY**	**SATURDAY**	**SUNDAY**
See pg. 34	See pg. 34	See pg. 34	See pg. 34
• Grated carrots dressed with lemon juice • Hanger steak on grated shallots (pg. 184) • Green beans • Custard with fructose	• White leek salad with vinaigrette (pg. 78) • Foies de volaille à la provençale (pg. 162) • Green salad • Cheese	• Zucchini mille feuille (pg. 82) • Squid à la provençale (pg. 122) • Compote à l'ancienne (pg. 235)	• Dill marinated salmon (pg. 98) • Confit of duck with apples (pg. 166) • Clafoutis aux framboises (pg. 246)
• Beef carpaccio • Green salad • Cheese	• Cabbage soup (cabbage, tomato, celery and fat-free chicken stock) • Steamed salmon filet • Broccoli • Poached pear CP	• Croque-aubergine (pg. 168) • Prune mousse (pg. 236)	• Endive gratin with ham (pg. 176) • Fruit

CP: carbohydrate-protein meal

WEEK 5

	Veal chops with two bell peppers (pg. 166)	Stuffed eggplants à la provençale (pg. 196)	Fruit zabaglione with almonds (pg. 240)
	MONDAY	**TUESDAY**	**WEDNESDAY**
Breakfast	See pg. 34	See pg. 34	See pg. 34
Lunch	• Cauliflower salad • Veal chops with two bell peppers (pg. 166) • Green salad • Cheese	• White leek salad with vinaigrette (pg. 78) • Trout with almonds • Broccoli • Curd cheese	• Spaghetti salad with mussels (pg. 80) • Entrecôte marchand de vin (pg. 178) • Sautéed endive • Fruit zabaglione with almonds (pg. 240)
Dinner	• Bell peppers stuffed with basmati rice (pg. 198) • Baked apple CP	• Stuffed eggplants à la provençale (pg. 196) • Yogurt	• Vegetarian stuffed tomatoes (pg. 204) • Fresh cheese CP

CP: carbohydrate-protein meal

Salmon tartare with fresh goat cheese (pg. 134)

Tomato and mozzarella millefeuille (pg. 90)

Vegetable omelet with chorizo (pg. 192)

Bavarois with berries (pg. 232)

THURSDAY	FRIDAY	SATURDAY	SUNDAY
See pg. 34	See pg. 34	See pg. 34	See pg. 34
• Avocado soup (pg. 64) • Salmon tartare with fresh goat cheese (pg. 134) • Green salad • Plain strawberries	• Tomato and mozzarella mille feuille (pg. 90) • Cheese omelet • Green salad • Yogurt	• Goat cheese mousse salad (pg. 76) • Pasque piperade (pg. 189) • Green salad • Cheese	• Southwest gourmet salad (pg. 81) • Poêlée de Saint-Jacques aux échalotes (pg. 120) • Bavarois with berries (pg. 232)
• Fried eggs • Ratatouille (pg. 212) • Fruit	• Spaghetti with basil tomato sauce (pg. 220) • Apple compote CP	• Vegetable omelet with chorizo (pg. 192) • Green salad • Cheese	• Tofu with green lentils (pg. 206) • Fruit

CP: carbohydrate-protein meal

WEEK 6

	Lentils	Leek quiche (pg. 102)	Foie gras sautéed with grapes (pg. 152)
	MONDAY	**TUESDAY**	**WEDNESDAY**
Breakfast	See pg. 34	See pg. 34	See pg. 34
Lunch	• Chick pea salad • Steak tartare • Green salad • Cheese	• Céleri rémoulade (celeriac, fat-free yogurt and mustard) • Veal liver seasoned with parsley • Peas • Yogurt	• Chilled broccoli soup (pg. 66) • Foie gras sautéed with grapes (pg. 152) • Salad • Cheese
Dinner	• Lentils with onions and tomato • Yogurt CP	• Leek quiche (pg. 102) • Green salad • Cheese	• Spaghetti with basil tomato sauce (pg. 220) • Apple compote CP

CP: carbohydrate-protein meal

Omelet andalouse (pg. 194)	Tofu skewers (pg. 200)	Cucumber and Prawn Mousse (pg. 62)	Chocolate mousse (pg. 230)
THURSDAY	**FRIDAY**	**SATURDAY**	**SUNDAY**
See pg. 34	See pg. 34	See pg. 34	See pg. 34
• Grated carrots dressed with vinaigrette • Chicken breast with curry (pg. 158) • Green salad • Fruit	• Endive salad with walnuts • Timbales de Saint-Jacques with prawns (pg. 114) • Sautéed fennel • Corsican fresh cheese cake (pg. 234)	• Cucumber and prawn mousse (pg. 62) • Chicken with apples (pg. 154) • Salad • Goat cheese	• Tuna tartare with aïoli (pg. 108) • Langoustines with leek fondue (pg. 112) • Chocolate mousse (pg. 230)
• Omelet andalouse (pg. 194) • Green salad • Plain strawberries	• Grated carrots dressed with lemon juice • Tofu skewers (pg. 200) • Yogurt CP	• Tuna with tomato and olives (pg. 142) • Salad • Custard with fructose	• Eggplant gratin with bacon cubes (pg. 174) • Baked apple

CP: carbohydrate-protein meal

WEEK 7

Tomato and mozzarella millefeuille (pg. 90)

Flan with peaches (pg. 226)

White leek salad with vinaigrette (pg. 78)

	MONDAY	TUESDAY	WEDNESDAY
Breakfast	See pg. 34	See pg. 34	See pg. 34
Lunch	• Tomato and mozzarella millefeuille (pg. 90) • Pork chop • Flageolet beans • Yogurt	• Red cabbage salad • Chicken livers sautéed in ginger (pg. 156) • Salad • Cheese	• White leek salad with vinaigrette (pg. 78) • Tuna filet with tomato (pg. 138) • Custard with fructose
Dinner	• Cabbage soup (cabbage, tomato, celery and fat-free chicken stock) • Egg whites poached in the soup or separately (2 or 3 per person) CP	• Greek salad (tomatoes + feta) • Cured ham • Flan with peaches (pg. 226)	• Green lentils • Basmati rice • Yogurt CP

CP: carbohydrate-protein meal

Canned tuna salad (pg. 74)	Salmon filets in foil parcels (pg. 140)	Omelet with eggplants (pg. 190)	Filet mignon skewers with prunes (pg. 182)
## THURSDAY	## FRIDAY	## SATURDAY	## SUNDAY
See pg. 34	See pg. 34	See pg. 34	See pg. 34
• Canned tuna salad (pg. 74) • Monkfish with champignons and red wine (pg. 137) • Salad • Cheese	• Asparagus dressed with vinaigrette • Salmon filets in foil parcels (pg. 140) • Fromage blanc drained	• Tomatoes with warm goat cheese (pg. 84) • Dorade à l'andalouse (pg. 136) • Plain raspberries	• Tuna stuffed avocado (pg. 96) • Filet mignon skewers with prunes (pg. 182) • Apricot cake (pg. 250)
• Zucchini stuffed with crab (pg. 126) • Clafoutis aux framboises (pg. 246)	• Spaghetti with champignon puree (1 fat-free yogurt and spices) • Cheese Raspberry coulis CP	• Omelet with eggplant (pg. 190) • Baked apple	• Vegetarian chili (pg. 202) • Fruit

CP: carbohydrate-protein meal

WEEK 8

	MONDAY	TUESDAY	WEDNESDAY
	montignac ratatouille (pg. 212)	Salmon tartare with fresh goat cheese (pg. 134)	Tomato and mozzarella millefeuille (pg. 90)
Breakfast	See pg. 34	See pg. 34	See pg. 34
Lunch	• Champignon salad • Grilled steak • Montignac ratatouille (keep to eat cold the next day) (pg. 212) • Apple	• Endive with bacon cubes (without croutons) • Salmon tartare with fresh goat cheese (pg. 134) • Salad • Plain raspberries	• Tomato and mozzarella millefeuille (pg. 90) • Veal chops with two bell peppers (pg. 166) • Green salad • Cheese
Dinner	• Bell peppers stuffed with basmati rice (pg. 198) • Yogurt CP	• Cold ratatouille (pg. 212) • Fried eggs • Peach in wine	• Spaghetti with basil tomato sauce (pg. 220) • Apple compote CP

CP: carbohydrate-protein meal

Trout with white wine (pg. 146)	Green lentil terrine (pg. 92)	Parfait with chocolate, raspberries and pistachios (pg. 238)	Peach soup with sweet wine (pg. 248)
THURSDAY	**FRIDAY**	**SATURDAY**	**SUNDAY**
See pg. 34	See pg. 34	See pg. 34	See pg. 34
• White leek salad with vinaigrette (pg. 78) • Trout with white wine (pg. 146) • Broccoli • Yogurt	• Green lentil terrine (pg. 92) • Bouillabaisse de l'Atlantique (pg. 127) • Salad • Cheese	• Quinoa à la provençale (pg. 100) • Hanger steak on grated shallots (pg. 184) • Green salad • Cheese	• Chilled cucumber soup with green apples (pg. 68) • Marinated scampi (pg. 116) • Peach soup with sweet wine (pg. 248)
• Vegetable soup (without potatoes) • Croque-aubergine (pg. 168) • Yogurt	• Basmati rice with tamari • Turkey ham • Poached pears CP	• Trout with white wine (pg. 146) • Parfait with chocolate, raspberries and pistachios (pg. 238)	• Whole-wheat tagliatelle with sauce bolognaise (pg. 218) • Fat-free soy cream fromage blanc

CP: carbohydrate-protein meal

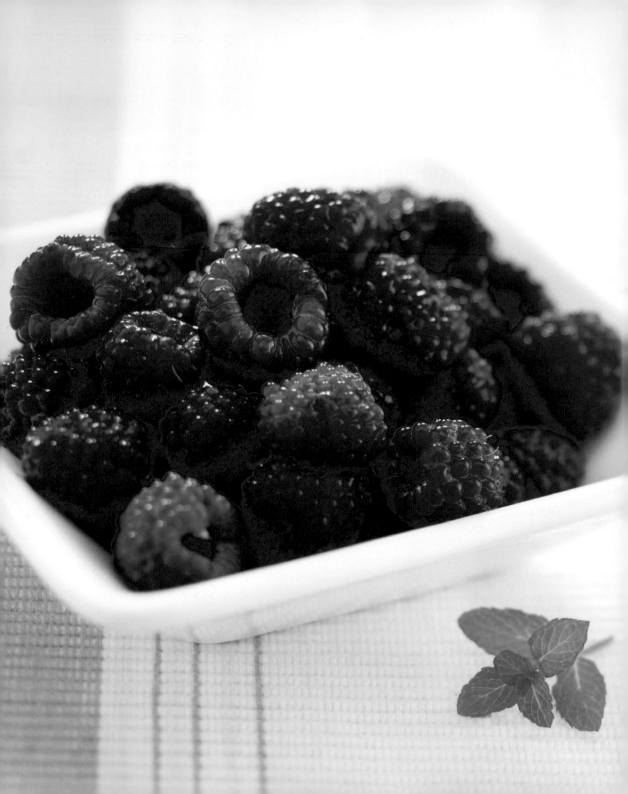

SPECIAL MENUS FOR WOMEN

Women who work, and for the most part cannot return home for lunch, always have a hard time finding something so they can eat properly where they work. Some of them have a company cafeteria, but despite the variety of dishes available, most of the proposed foods are of a mediocre quality and above all cooked using industrial processes which are contrary to the recommendations of the Montignac method (keeping them warm for a long time, use of bad fats, etc.).

This is why many women rightly prefer using a lunch box, i.e. bringing their meal to work with them, after carefully preparing it at home.

Aside from the fact that this solution is much cheaper than eating in the cafeteria, it offers a better way of managing a food balance throughout the day, and preventing last minute improvisation.

This solution also makes it possible in all cases to make better food choices based on weight goals, whether they involve not gaining weight or losing weight.

The table below contains an example of menus for a week of balanced eating which is in line with women's preferences:

• more fish than meat;

• more white meat than red meat;

• various vegetables (raw and cooked), as well as good carbohydrates (low glycemic index).

GOOD TO KNOW

These lunch meals have the advantage of being able to be eaten cold or hot, based on the possibility of reheating at the workplace. They are rich in proteins, since carbohydrates dominate in the dinner menus. As always in the Montignac method, the good fats are in the vast majority (olive oil and omega-3)

SPECIAL MENUS FOR WOMEN

	Spaghetti with basil tomato sauce (pg. 220)	Quinoa tabouli (pg. 72)	plain raspberry
	MONDAY	**TUESDAY**	**WEDNESDAY**
Breakfast	See pg. 34	See pg. 34	See pg. 34
Lunch	• Tomato salad • Steamed chicken breast • Broccoli • Yogurt	• Cucumber with soy cream. • Steamed salmon filet • Chick peas • Apple	• Grated carrots dressed with lemon juice • Sliced turkey • Green lentils • Plain raspberries
Dinner	• Spaghetti with basil tomato sauce (pg. 220) • Apple compote CP	• Quinoa tabouli (pg. 72) • Yogurt	• Cabbage soup (cabbage, tomato, celery and fat-free chicken stock) • 2 poached egg whites • Yogurt

CP: carbohydrate-protein meal

montignac ratatouille (pg. 212)	Lentils	Vegetarian chili (pg. 202)	tian à la provencale (pg. 214)
## THURSDAY	## FRIDAY	## SATURDAY	## SUNDAY
See pg. 34	See pg. 34	See pg. 34	See pg. 34
• Red cabbage salad • Hard boiled egg • Montignac ratatouille (pg. 212) • Plain strawberries	• Céleri rémoulade (celeriac, fat-free yogurt and mustard) • Water-packed tuna • Green beans • Custard with fructose	• Avocado dressed with vinaigrette • Stuffed eggplants à la provençale (pg. 196) • Green salad • Cheese • Baked apple	• Greek salad (tomatoes + feta) • Dorade à l'andalouse (pg. 136) • Tian à la provençale (pg. 214) • Goat cheese cake (pg. 242)
• Quinoa à la provençale (pg. 100) • Soy cream fromage blanc	• Green lentils and basmati rice • Yogurt	• Vegetarian chili (pg. 202) • Compote à l'ancienne (pg. 235)	• Leek quiche (pg. 102) • Green salad • Peach in wine

CP: carbohydrate-protein meal

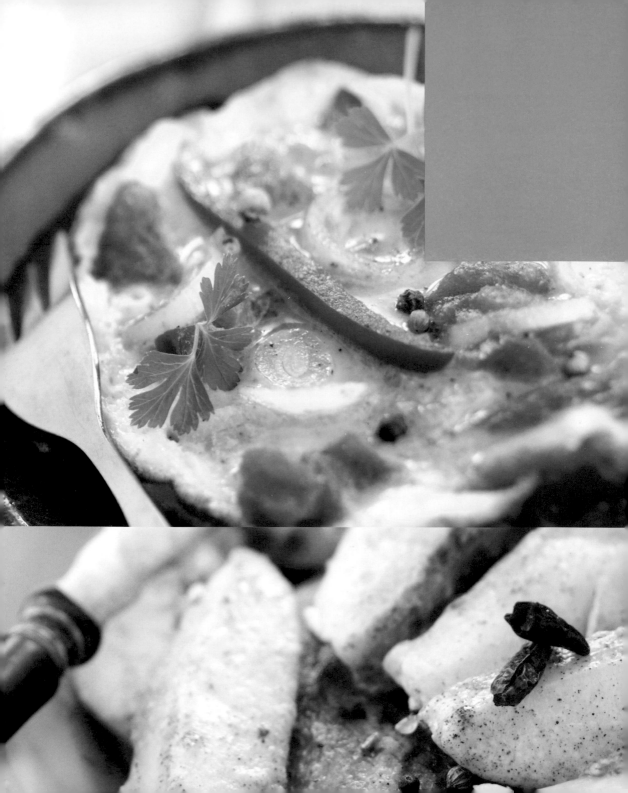

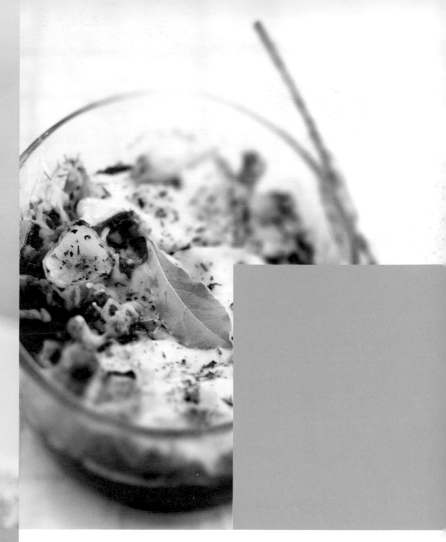

100
RECIPES

All the recipes are compatibles with Montignac method phase I. They are simple and easy to make.
Most of them take no more than 15 to 20 minutes of preparation.

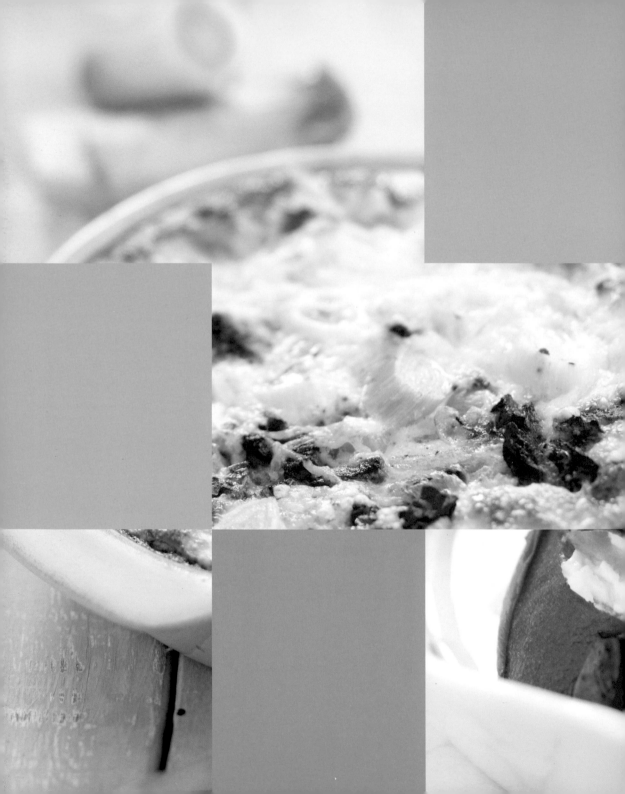

APPETIZERS

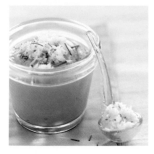

Cream of avocado soup with crab

Serves 4

■ **Preparation time:**
20 minutes

■ **Refrigeration time:**
1 hour

■ **Ingredients:**
> 3 ripe avocados
> Juice of 1 lime
> 1 small shallot
> 2 tablespoons of low-fat crème fraîche (or soy cream)
> 1 tablespoon of tomato paste
> 1 drop of Worcestershire sauce
> 18fl oz (50 cl) of fat-free cold chicken stock
> 1 pinch of Cayenne pepper
> 7oz (200 g) canned crab
> Paprika
> 4 small spring onions with their green parts (for garnish)
> Salt and pepper

Cut the avocados in half. Remove the pit and place the flesh in the bowl of a mixer. Add the lime juice and mix until it is creamy and smooth.

Chop the shallot and add it to the mixer's bowl with the crème fraîche, the tomato paste, the Worcestershire sauce and chicken stock. Add the Cayenne pepper, salt and pepper. Mix until the soup is smooth. Chill for 1 hour.

Drain the crab and remove any cartilage if necessary.

To serve, pour the chilled soup and add the bits of crab. Sprinkle lightly with paprika and arrange the onions on top.

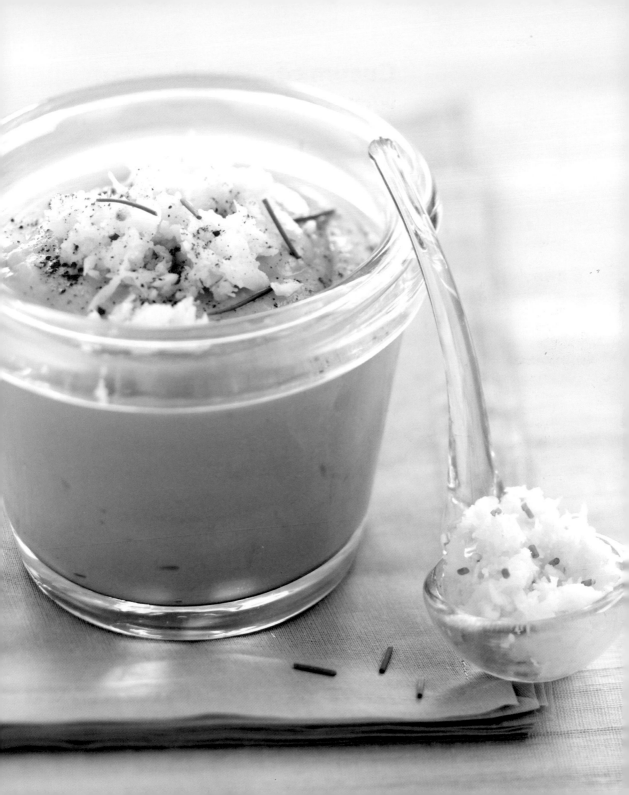

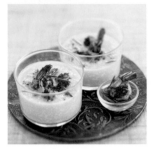

Cucumber and Prawn Mousse

Serves 4

■ **Preparation time:**
20 minutes

■ **Ingredients:**
> 2 large cucumbers
> 2 chopped shallots
> 18fl oz (50 cl) of fat-free cold chicken stock
> 14fl oz (40 cl) soy cream (or low-fat crème fraîche)
> 16 medium-sized cooked prawns
> 1 teaspoon of paprika
> 1 small bunch of chives
> Salt and pepper

Peel the cucumbers. Cut them into four lengthwise and remove the middle with the seeds. Chop roughly. Put them in the mixer with the chopped shallots.

Add the chicken stock and the low-fat crème fraîche (or soy cream), and season. Mix this again until it becomes smooth. Chill.

Peel the prawns and roll them in plenty of paprika.

Chop the chives before serving. Mix the soup again to make it very smooth. Pour it into individual bowls. Arrange the prawns on top. Sprinkle a little paprika and add the chives.

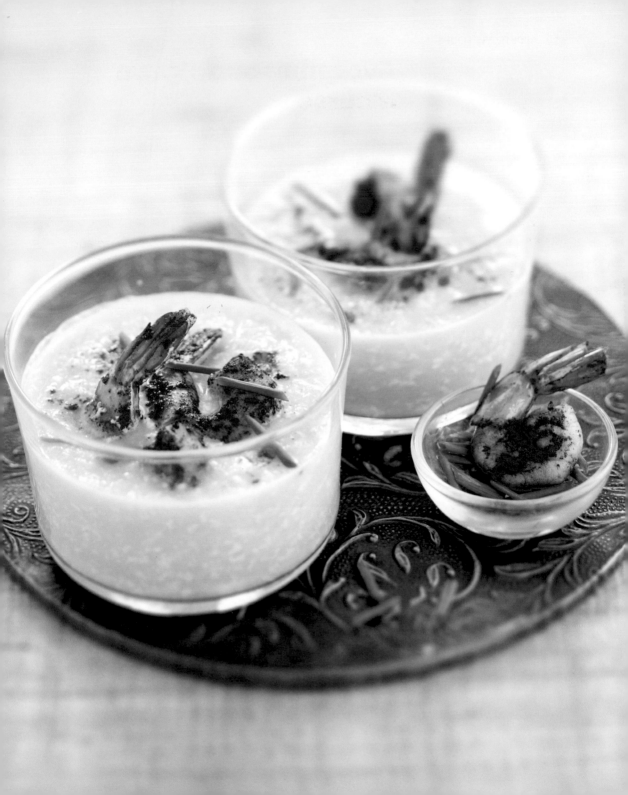

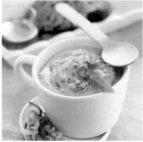

Avocado soup

Serves 4

■ **Preparation time:**
10 minutes
■ **Cooking time:**
5 minutes

■ **Ingredients:**
> 2 ripe avocados
> Juice of ½ lemon
> 1 large chopped onion
> 1 tablespoon of olive oil
> 9fl oz (25 cl) soy cream
(or low-fat crème fraîche)
> A few basil leaves
> Salt and pepper

Use a small spoon to remove the avocado flesh. Sprinkle with lemon juice to keep it from turning brown.
Use a fork to completely mash. Set aside.

Sauté the onion in olive oil in a frying pan. Season with salt and pepper.

Add the avocado puree and let it simmer over a few low flame until obtaining a smooth cream.

Let cool. Pour in the soy cream.

Serve chilled and decorate the plate or bowl with a few basil leaves.

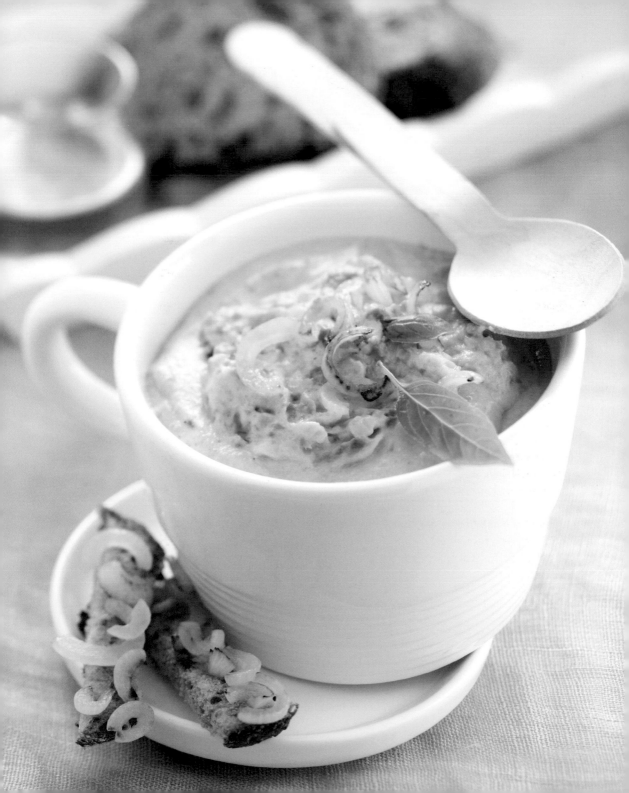

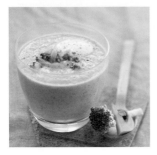

Chilled broccoli soup

Serves 4

■ **Preparation time:**
20 minutes
■ **Cooking time:**
15 minutes
■ **Refrigeration time:**
2 hours

■ **Ingredients:**
> 1 large onion
> 2 tablespoons of olive oil
> 18fl oz (50 cl) of fat-free
cold chicken stock
> Heads of broccoli
> 1 box of chopped chives
> 2oz (50 g) of canned
champignon mushrooms
> 7fl oz (20 cl) soy cream
(or low-fat crème fraîche)
> A few walnut halves
> Grated nutmeg
> Salt and pepper

Chop the onion and sauté it in olive oil in a pot until soft.

Add the stock and bring to a boil.

Cut the broccoli into small pieces and add to the pot. Cook uncovered over a medium flame for 5 minutes.

When done cooking, add the chopped chives and champignons. Season with salt and pepper.

Mix all the ingredients in a mixer until smooth. Chill for at least 2 hours.

Right before serving, mix in the soy cream and add the walnuts and little grated nutmeg.

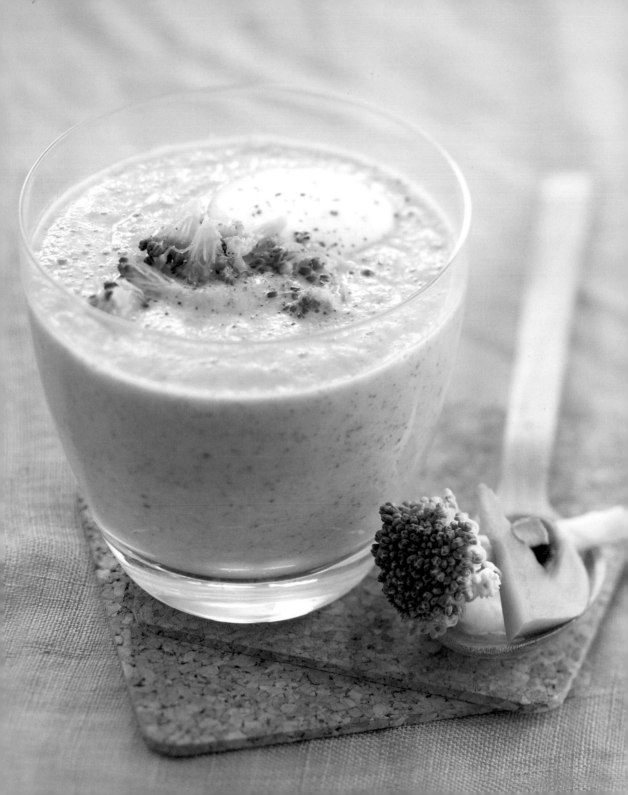

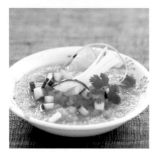

Chilled cucumber soup with green apples

Serves 4

■ **Preparation time:**
15 minutes
■ **Refrigeration time:**
5 hours

■ **Ingredients:**
> 5 Granny Smith apples
> 2 cucumbers
> 1 organic lime
> 5 small chopped white onions
> 1 fennel stalk
> 8 sprigs of fresh coriander
> 2 sprigs of dill
> 3 tablespoons of extra virgin olive oil
> 2 or 3 pinches of Cayenne pepper
> Salt and pepper

Peel the apples. Cut into quarters and remove the cores.

Peel the cucumbers. Cut into quarters and remove the middle (seeds). Chop into lengths.

Remove 8 nice lime zests. Squeeze the lime to obtain the juice.

Put the quartered apples, cucumber lengths, chopped onions, fennel stalk, coriander, lime juice, dill sprigs, olive oil and Cayenne pepper in the bowl of a mixer. Mix until obtaining a uniform liquid puree. Season with salt and pepper.

Chill for at least 5 hours.

Serve decorating with the lime zest and the rest of the herbs used for the recipe. Drizzle with olive oil.

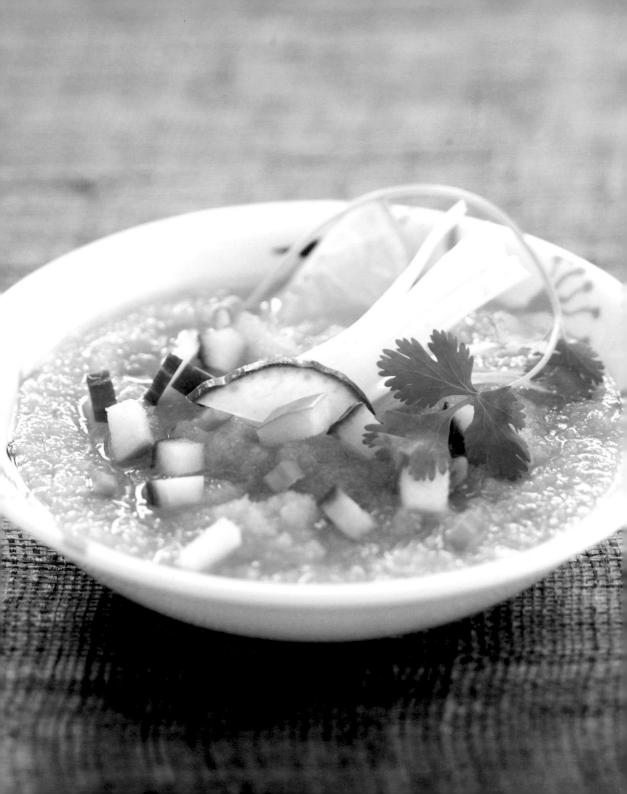

Salade landaise

Serves 4

■ **Preparation time:**
20 minutes
■ **Cooking time:**
15 minutes

■ **Ingredients:**
> 1 small jar of gésiers
confits
> 3½ oz (100 g) of
lamb's lettuce
> 3¾ oz (110 g) of
spinach leaves
> 4 large champignons
> 4 fresh figs
> 3½ oz (100 g) of
half-cooked foie gras
> 1 packet of sliced
smoked duck breast
> 3½ oz (100 g) of
prosciutto chiffonnade
> 2oz (50 g) of pine nuts
> 1 bunch of chervil
> Vinaigrette made from olive
oil and balsamic vinegar
(see pg. 78)

Open the jar of gésiers confits. Remove the fat with paper towels or heat it in an oven at 100°C for 15 minutes.

Sort the lamb's lettuce and wash carefully to remove the
sand. Wash the spinach leaves. Dry. Set aside.

Wash and dry the champignons. Remove the dirty end.
Peel them and slice.

Arrange the salad on 4 plates. Cut the figs in quarters
and place them on the lamb's lettuce and on the champignons.

Cut the foie gras into small slices using a sharp knife.
Arrange it on the plates dividing uniformly: the foie
gras, duck breast, gésiers, prosciutto chiffonnade, pine
nuts and shredded chervil.

Pour the vinaigrette on the salad (one and half tablespoons per plate).

Salade d'épinards
à la sévillane

Serves 4

Preparation time:
25 minutes

Cooking time:
10 minutes

Ingredients:
> 2¼ lb (1 kg) of fresh spinach
> A little olive oil
> 4 minced garlic cloves
> 1 teaspoon of mild paprika
> 1 teaspoon of powdered cumin
> 12oz (350 g) of cooked chick peas (save some of the cooking water)
> A few drops of balsamic vinegar
> 2 chopped hard-boiled eggs
> Salt and pepper

Prepare the spinach: remove the stalks from the leaves and chop them. Boil for 30 seconds and drain in a strainer.

Heat some olive oil in a pot and sauté the minced garlic. Add the paprika and cumin. Mix well.

Add the spinach and the chick peas, then sprinkle a few drops of vinegar and a little of the cooking water from the chick peas.

Cook for 3 to 5 minutes, constantly stirring. Season with salt and pepper.

Serve in small individual saucepans.

Drizzle with olive oil and decorate with chopped hard-boiled eggs.

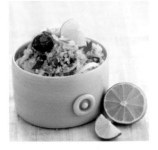

Quinoa tabouli

Serves 4

Preparation time:
20 minutes
Standing time:
25 minutes
Cooking time:
4 minutes

Ingredients:
> 3½ oz (100 g) quinoa
> 3 bunches Italian parsley
> 1 bunch of fresh mint
> 4 tomatoes on a vine
> 3 spring onions with
their stalk
> Juice of 3 limes
> 4 tablespoons of olive oil
> Salt and pepper

Place the quinoa in a fine strainer. Rinse it under plenty of running water. Put two times its volume of water in a pan. Add salt. Bring to a boil. Cook covered for 3 minutes. Remove from the flame and let it 10 minutes to absorb the water. Drain in a strainer.

Wash the parsley and the mint. Shred, dry and chop them very finely.

Drop the tomatoes into boiling water and cook for 40 seconds then rinse under cold water. Remove their skin. Cut into quarters and deseed. Chop the pulp with a knife.

Chop the onions and their stalks very finely.

Pour the lime juice into a salad bowl. Dissolve a little salt in it. Whisk with the olive oil. Add the well-drained quinoa and mix. Let sit for 15 minutes.

Add the parsley, mint, tomatoes, onions, season with pepper and mix.

★ This tabouli can be served immediately or chilled after having covered the top of the salad bowl with plastic wrap.

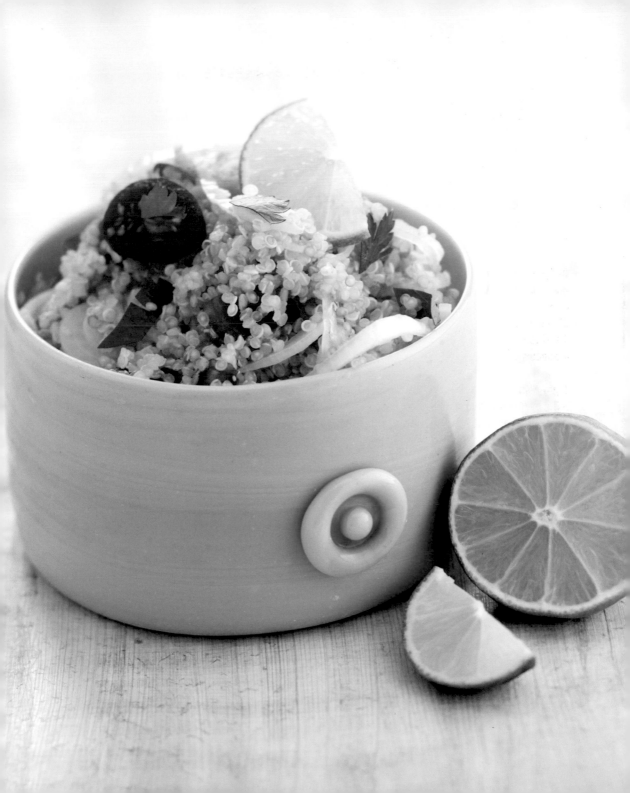

Canned tuna salad

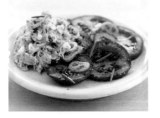

Serves 4

■ **Preparation time:**
20 minutes
■ **Cooking time:**
10 minutes

■ **Ingredients:**
> 2 eggs + 1 yolk
> 3 shallots
> 7oz (200 g) canned
water packed tuna
> 1 tablespoon of
strong Dijon mustard
> 4 tablespoons of olive oil
> Juice of 1 lemon
> 2 tablespoons of
chopped chives
> 5fl oz (15 cl) soy cream
(or low-fat crème fraîche)
> Salt and pepper

Hard boil the eggs for ten minutes. Cool them in cold water and then peel. Chop them finely.

Peel the shallots and chop finely.

Drain the tuna and then mash it with a fork.

In a large salad bowl, add the mustard, egg yolk and olive oil. Whisk as if making mayonnaise. Add the mashed tuna, the hard boiled eggs, lemon juice, shallots, chives and soy cream. Season with salt and pepper. Mix and chill until mealtime.

Serve on a bed of lettuce or tomato slices.

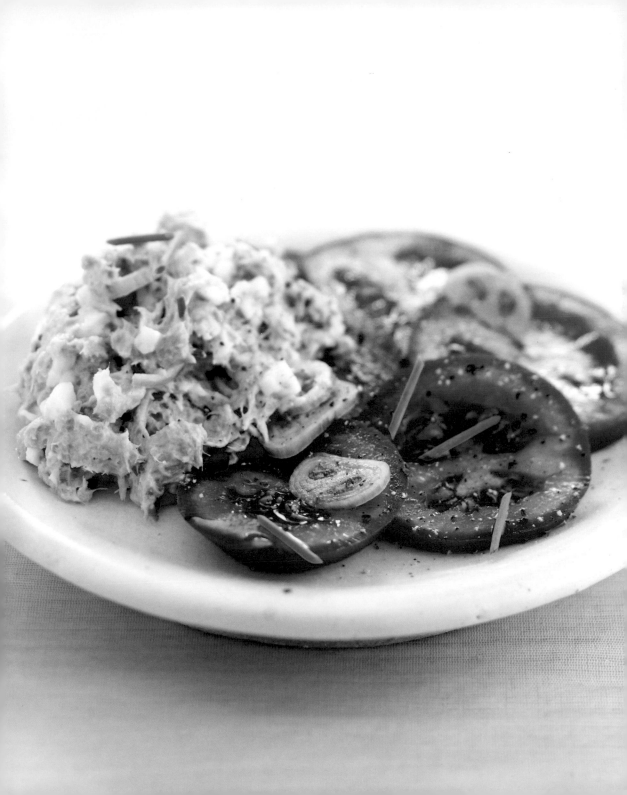

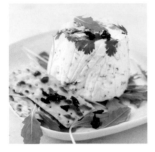

Goat cheese mousse salad

Serves 4

Preparation time:
20 minutes

Refrigeration time:
2 hours

Ingredients:
> 12oz (350 g) of fresh goat cheese
> 9fl oz (50 cl) of very cold liquid crème fraîche (whipping cream)
> Various lettuces and herbs: arugula, spinach leaves, chervil, Italian parsley, tarragon, etc.
> 4fl oz (12 cl) olive oil
> Vinaigrette (olive oil and balsamic vinegar, see pg. 78)
> 2 teaspoons of tapenade
> Salt and freshly ground pepper

Drain the goat cheese well in a strainer

Whip the crème fraîche until stiff. Chill.

Wash and sort the lettuce and herbs.

In a large bowl, mix the goat cheese and olive oil with an electric beater. Season with salt and pepper. Mix until obtaining a uniform cream.

Add gently to the whipped crème fraîche with a spatula.

Oil 4 deep ramekins with olive oil and fill with the mixture. Chill for 2 hours.

When serving place the salad on individual plates. Dress with 1 or 2 teaspoons of vinaigrette.

Unmold the ramekins by turning them over sharply on the center of each place.

Dilute the tapenade in 1 or 2 tablespoons of olive oil and uniformly drizzle over the top of each goat cheese mousse; grind fresh black pepper over the top.

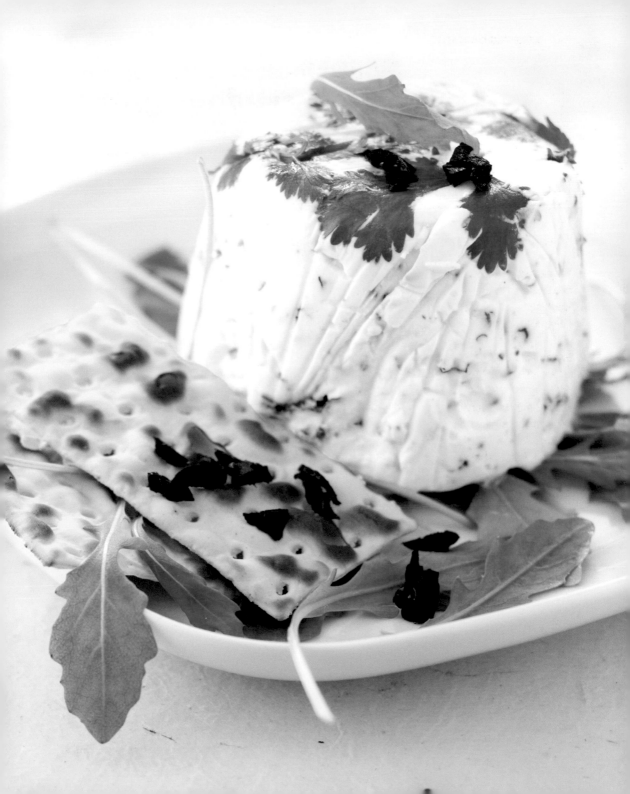

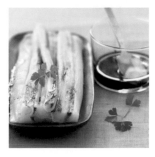

White leek salad with vinaigrette

Serves 4

■ **Preparation time:**
5 minutes
■ **Cooking time:**
40 minutes
■ **Refrigeration time:**
1 hour

■ **Ingredients:**
> 8 leeks, white part
> 2 bunches of Italian parsley
(for decoration)

■ **For the vinaigrette**
> 1 teaspoon of strong
mustard
> 1 tablespoon of balsamic
vinegar
> 4 tablespoons of olive oil
> ¼ tablespoon of garlic
powder
> Salt and pepper

Remove the roots and white bottoms of the leeks. Remove the first leaf which often contains sand, then wash carefully.

Put a large pinch of salt in a pan full of water. Drop in the leeks and cook over a medium flame for 40 minutes. Drain, let cool and chill for at least 1 hour.

Prepare the vinaigrette.

Before serving, cut the leeks in two lengthwise. Dry them with paper towels. Arrange them on individual plates. Dress with vinaigrette and garnish with parsley.

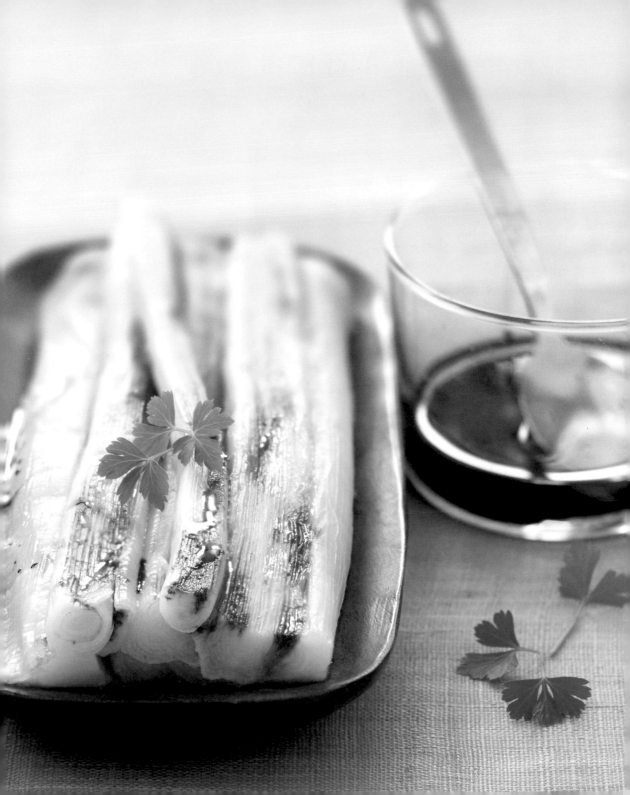

Spaghetti salad with mussels

Serves 4

✳ To prepare the day before

◾ **Preparation time:**
20 minutes
◾ **Cooking time:**
15 minutes

◾ **Ingredients:**
> 9oz (250 ml) spaghetti
cooked *al dente* (cook the
night before)
> 2 tablespoons of olive oil
> 2¼ lb (1 kg) of cultivated
mussels
> 4 chopped shallots
> 7fl oz (20 cl) dry
white wine
> 1 bunch Italian parsley
> Pepper

◾ **For the vinaigrette**
> 3 tablespoons of olive oil
> 1/2 tablespoon of
balsamic vinegar
> 1 pinch of curry
> Salt and pepper

The night before cook the spaghetti in a pot of slightly salted boiling water, only for 5 minutes. Drain, then let cool in a salad bowl and mix with 1 tablespoon of olive oil so they don't stick. Set aside for the night.

Carefully scrape and trim the mussels. Sauté the shallots in a large pan with a little olive oil. Season with pepper. Add the white wine and bring to a boil for 1 minute.

Add the mussels and cook covered for 3 to 5 minutes until they open completely. Put them in a strainer and let them cool under cold water. Prepare the vinaigrette.

Remove the mussels from their shells.

Divide the spaghetti into soup plates. Arrange the mussels on top. Dress with vinaigrette and garnish with parsley.

✳ Keeping the pasta in the refrigerator overnight decreases the glycemic index enough so that it becomes a phase I food.

Southwest gourmet salad

Serves 4

■ **Preparation time:**
15 minutes
■ **Cooking time:**
10 minutes

■ **Ingredients:**
> 11oz (300 g) fresh
string beans
> 3½ oz (100 g) of fresh
champignons
> Juice of 1 lemon
> 20 slices of smoked duck
breast
> 1 small can of anchovy
filets in olive oil
> 2oz (50 g) of pine nuts
> 2oz (50 g) of fresh
chopped chives
> 4 bunches of Italian parsley
(for decoration)

■ **For the vinaigrette**
> 1 teaspoon of strong Dijon
mustard
> 1 tablespoon of balsamic
vinegar
> 2 minced garlic cloves
> 3 tablespoons of olive oil
> Salt and pepper

String the string beans: remove the ends and any strings. Cut them in half. Bring 2 liters of water to boil in a pan. Drop in the string beans and let them cook over a medium flame for 10 minutes. Drain and put them in very cold water. Drain again. Dry them with paper towels if necessary.

Remove the dirty end of the champignons. Wash, drain and dry them. Cut into thin slices. Quickly sprinkle with lemon juice to keep them from turning brown.

Make the vinaigrette in the bottom of a large salad bowl. Mix the mustard in the balsamic vinegar. Add the minced garlic and olive oil. Season with salt and pepper. Add the string beans and champignons. Mix well to coat well with the vinaigrette.

Divide the contents of the salad bowl on four large plates. Add the slices of smoked duck breast, the anchovies and pine nuts. Sprinkle with chopped chives and garnish with parsley.

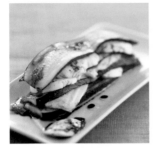

Zucchini millefeuille

Serves 4

■ **Preparation time:**
15 minutes

■ **Cooking time:**
8 minutes

■ **Ingredients:**
> 2 large zucchini
> 8 tablespoons of olive oil
> 3 mozzarella balls
> 2 garlic cloves
> 1 tablespoon of balsamic vinegar
> 1 pinch of herbes de Provence
> Salt and pepper

Rinse and drain the zucchini. Cut them in half and eliminate the ends. Cut them into thin 0.5 cm slices lengthwise.

In a large frying pan, pour in half the olive oil and brown the zucchini slices over a medium flame. Dry them with paper towels.

Drain the mozzarella. Cut it into thin slices, season with salt and pepper.

Peel and press the garlic cloves.

In a bowl, mix the balsamic vinegar, the rest of the olive oil and the pressed garlic. Season with salt and pepper.

Create a millefeuille by alternating slices of zucchini and mozzarella.

Sprinkle with sauce and a pinch of herbes de Provence.

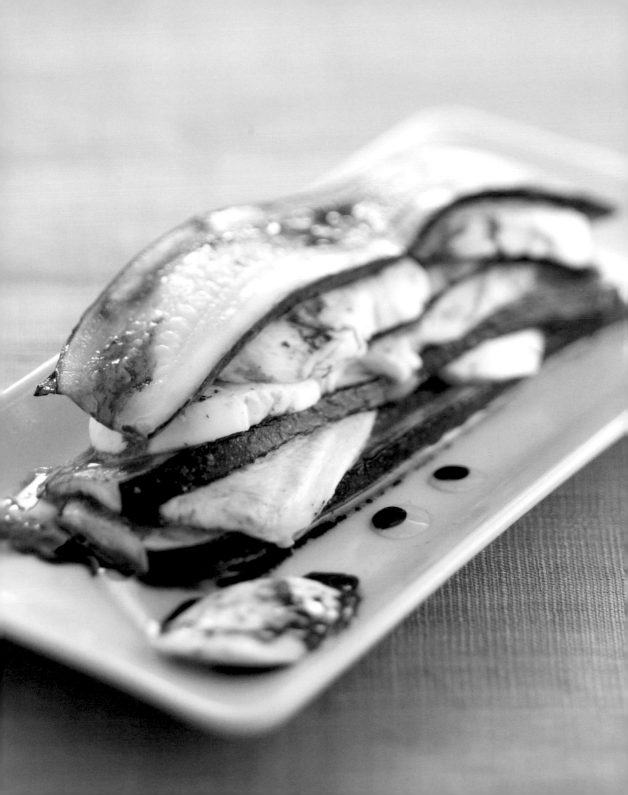

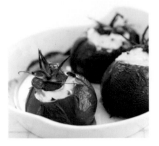

Tomatoes with warm goat cheese

Serves 4

■ **Preparation time:**
10 minutes
■ **Cooking time:**
45 minutes

■ **Ingredients:**
> 8 medium size tomatoes
> 11oz (300 g) of fresh goat cheese (2 to 3)
> 4 tablespoons of olive oil
> A few basil leaves
(for the garnish)
> Salt and pepper

Preheat the oven to 180°C.

Wash the tomatoes and then cut the top off with a sharp knife. Carefully remove the interior with a small spoon. Turn the tomatoes over and let them drain well.

In a bowl mix the fresh goat cheese with olive oil until obtaining a uniform paste. Season with salt and pepper.

Fill the tomatoes. Put the top back on and place on a baking dish. Bake 40 to 45 minutes.

Serve hot on a bed of lettuce garnished with basil leaves.

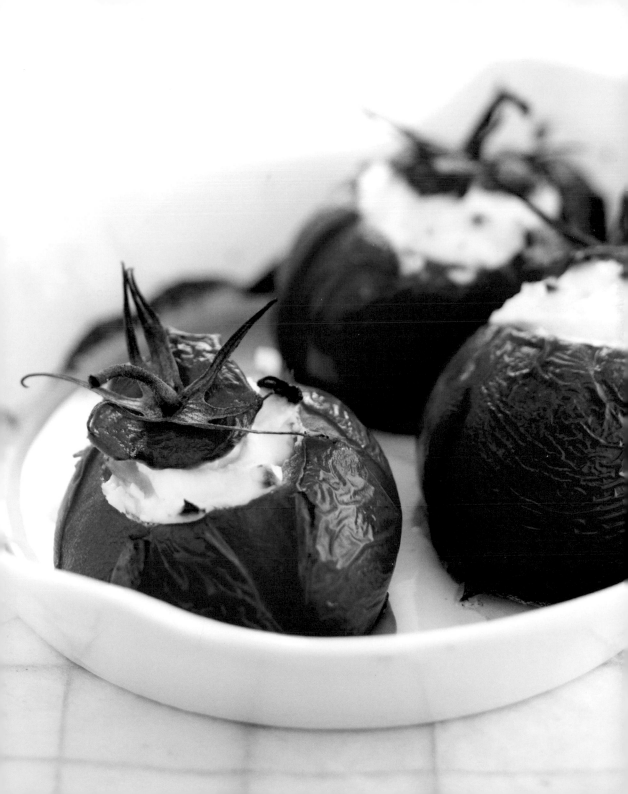

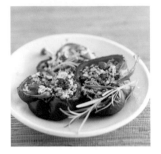

Bell peppers stuffed with ewe cheese

Serves 4

■ **Preparation time:**
20 minutes
■ **Cooking time:**
45 minutes

■ **Ingredients:**
> 4 red bell peppers
> 4 small tomatoes
> 3 chopped shallots
> 4 tablespoons of olive oil
> 3 minced garlic cloves
> 3½ oz (100 g) pitted
green olives
> 3½ oz (100 g) pitted
black olives
> 11oz (300 g) of fresh ewe
cheese
> 1 tablespoon of chopped
parsley
> 1 teaspoon of fresh thyme
> Salt and pepper

Preheat the oven to 200 °C.

Cut the bell peppers in half lengthwise and clean out the insides.

Boil the tomatoes for 30 seconds. Put them under cold water, then peel and deseed them and cut into small pieces.

Sauté the shallots with 2 tablespoons of olive oil in a frying pan. Add the garlic at the end of cooking.

Chop the green and black olives.

In a bowl, mash the cheese with 1 tablespoon of olive oil. Add the tomatoes, shallots, garlic, olives, parsley and thyme. Season with salt and pepper.

Fill the peppers.

Oil a baking dish, put the bell peppers on it and bake 35 minutes, even longer for softer bell peppers.

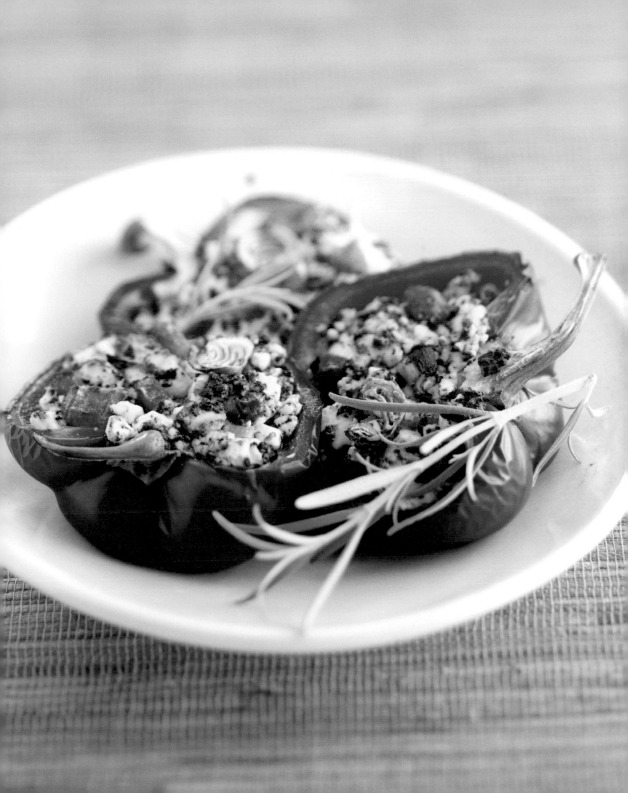

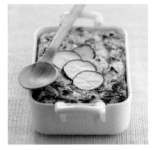

Gratin de courgette à la grecque

Serves 4

▉ **Preparation time:**
15 minutes
▉ **Cooking time:**
55 minutes
▉ **Standing time:**
30 minutes

▉ **Ingredients:**
> 2½ lb (1.25 kg) of zucchini
> 7oz (200 g) feta cheese
> 3 eggs
> 2oz (60 g) grated
parmesan
> Olive oil
(for the baking dish)
> Salt and pepper

Wash the zucchini and then cut off the ends. Cook them whole in salted boiling water for around 15 minutes, then drain them.

Mash the warm zucchini and let them sit for 30 minutes in a strainer to drain well.

Mash the feta with a fork.

Scramble the eggs in a salad bowl. Add the mashed feta and grated parmesan. Season with salt and pepper and mix well.

Add the zucchini to the mixture.

Pour the mixture into an oiled baking dish. Bake at 160°C for 40 minutes. The top of the gratin needs to be browned.

✳ This can also be used as a side dish.

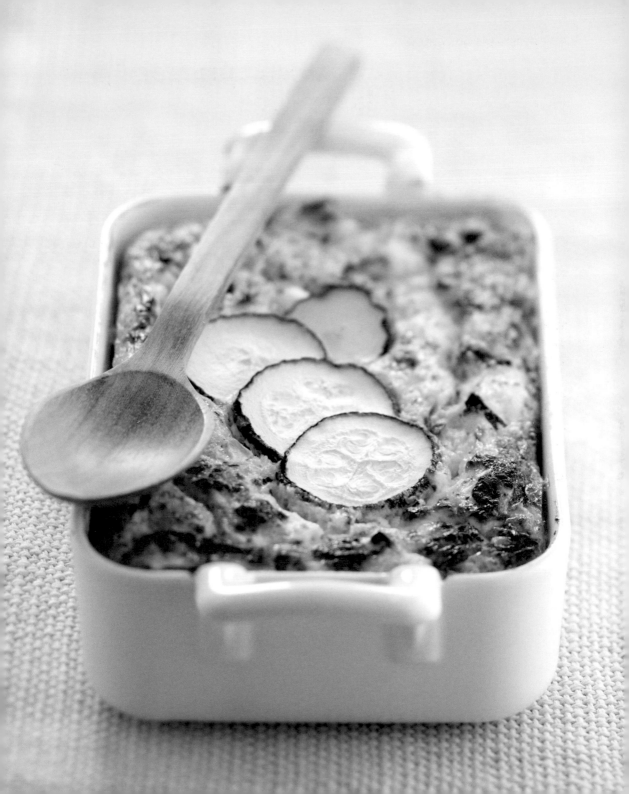

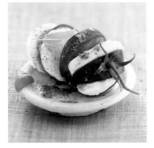

Tomato and mozzarella millefeuille

Serves 4

■ **Preparation time:**
5 minutes

■ **Ingredients:**
> 4 large tomatoes
> 2 mozzarella balls
> 1 small jar of pesto
> 2 tablespoons of olive oil
> A few fresh basil leaves
> Salt and pepper

Wash the tomatoes, then drain and dry them well. Cut each tomato into 4 horizontal slices. Put them on paper towels to absorb most of the moisture.

Cut the mozzarella into 12 slices.

Rebuild the 4 tomatoes placing pesto, mozzarella and salt and pepper between each slice.

Drizzle with olive oil and garnish with basil.

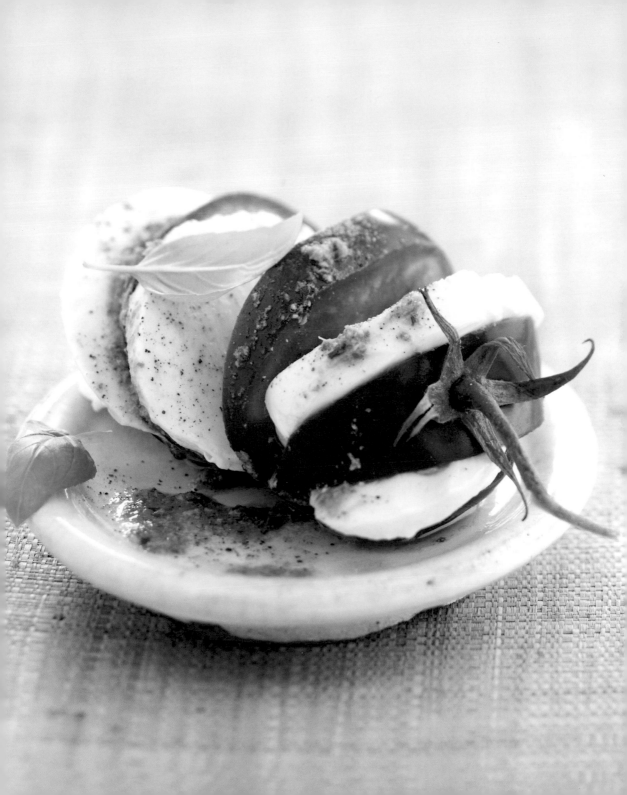

Green lentil terrine

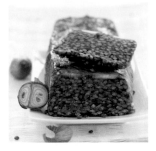

Serves 6

Preparation time:
15 minutes
Cooking time:
1 hour
Soaking time:
1 hour
Refrigeration time:
5 hour

Ingredients:
> 4oz (125 g) Du Puy
green lentils
> 1 chopped onion
> Thyme, bay leaf
> 4 gelatin leaves
> 2 tomatoes
> 1 tablespoon of
chopped chives

For the vinaigrette
> 1 teaspoon of
Dijon mustard
> 1 tablespoon
of Xérès vinegar
> 3 tablespoons of olive oil
> 1 chopped shallot
> 1 tablespoon of
chopped parsley
> Salt and pepper

Let the lentils soak for an hour in cold water.

In one liter of salted water cook the chopped onion,
thyme and bay leaf for 25 minutes.
Put the cooking water through a conical strainer.
Add the lentils to the water and cook until they are soft
(30 to 40 minutes).

Soak the gelatin leaves in cold water to soften them.

Eliminate two thirds of the lentil cooking water. Drain
the gelatin leaves and add them to the lentils. Put the
mixture into a terrine previously covered with plastic
wrap. Chill for at least 5 hours.

Prepare the vinaigrette in a bowl: mix the mustard and
vinegar, add the olive oil and then the chopped shallot
and parsley and season with salt and pepper.

Cut the terrine into thin slices. Garnish with large tomato
chunks and chopped chives. Dress with vinaigrette.

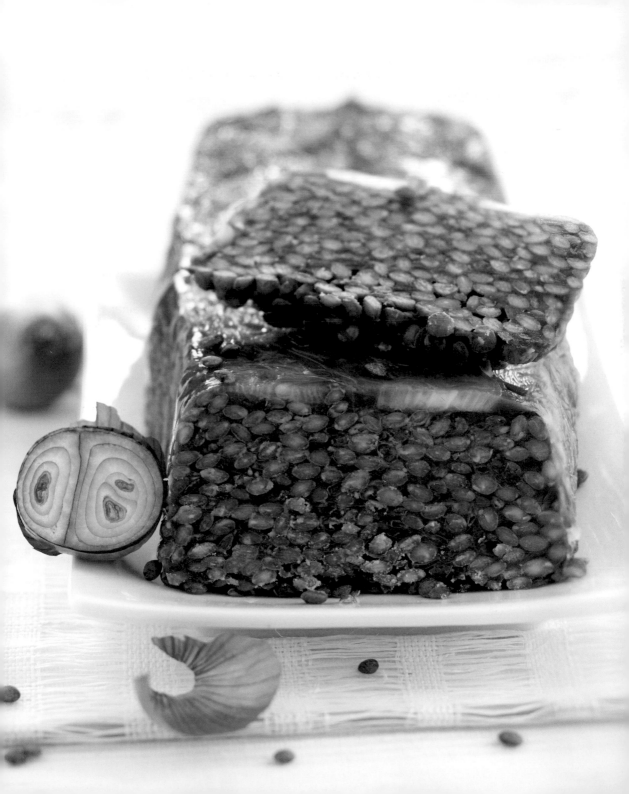

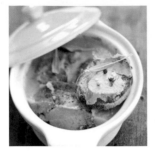

Foie gras terrine

Serves 6

✱ To do the night before

◼ **Preparation time:**
1 hour
◼ **Cooking time:**
1 hour
◼ **Refrigeration time:**
36 hours

◼ **Ingredients:**
> 3¼ lb (1.5 kg) foie gras (raw)
> 1½ tea spoon (7 g) fine salt
> ½ tea spoon (2 g) pepper
> 1 tablespoon of allspice
> 1 pinch of grated nutmeg
(optional)
> 4fl oz (10 cl) of armagnac
or cognac

Take the foie gras out of the refrigerator at least 2 hours ahead of time so that it is at a good temperature for being handled without breaking. Rinse it to remove any traces of blood. Dry.
Gently spread the two lobes to remove the nerves: gently pull the nerves without breaking using the tip of a potato peeler. You can make cuts to find the path of the veins and nerves. Separate the two lobes if this was not done when removing the nerves.
In a bowl mix the salt, pepper, allspice, nutmeg and armagnac well to create a marinade.
Place the lobes in a bowl brush them with plenty of marinade on all surfaces for 5 minutes so the marinade penetrates. Let it sit in the bottom of the bowl in the rest of the marinade. Place plastic film on the container to seal it well and chill over night in the refrigerator.
Take the liver out of the refrigerator two hours before preparing the terrine. Put the lobes into a terrine and starting with the bigger one (convex part on the top), pressing down as much as possible so that there are no holes.
Preheat the oven to 110 °C without the fan. Boil the water. When the oven is preheated, place the terrine in the middle of a baking dish, fill the dish with the boiling water up to the middle of the terrine and cook for around 50 to 60 minutes.
Let the terrine cool. When it has returned to room temperature, put it in the refrigerator with a cover or plastic wrap and let it sit at least 24 hours before tasting.

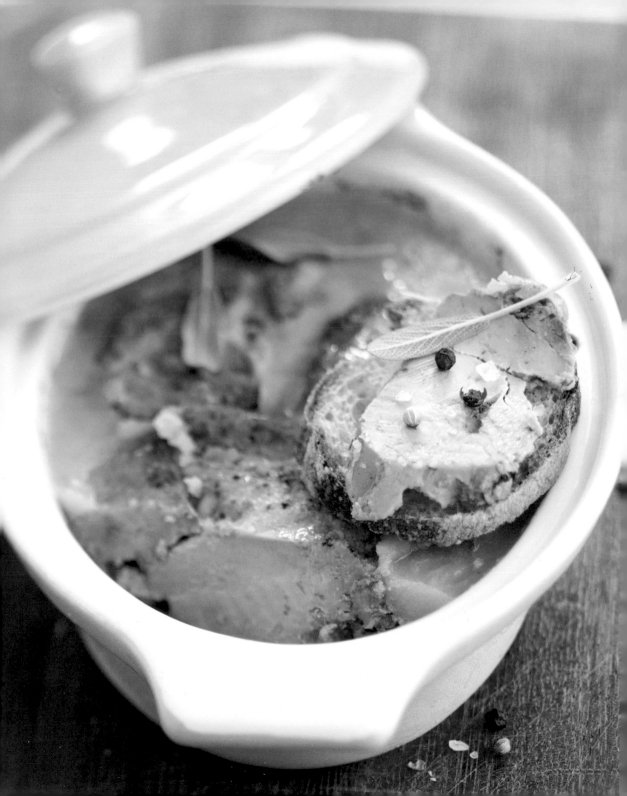

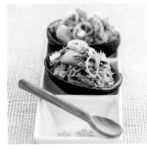

Tuna stuffed avocados

Serves 4

■ **Preparation time:**
15 minutes
■ **Refrigeration time:**
1 hour

■ **Ingredients:**
> 1 small celery stalk
> 1 small can of water
packed tuna 5oz (150 g)
> 1 hard boiled egg
> 2 large ripe avocados
> Juice of 1 lime
> 1 chopped shallot
> 2 tablespoons of
mayonnaise made
with olive oil
> 4 or 5 chopped black olives
> Salt and pepper

Remove the strings from the celery and chop finely.

Drain the tuna and then crumble it.

Finely chop the egg.

Cut the avocados in half, remove the pit and sprinkle immediately with lemon juice to keep them from turning brown.

Remove the pulp from the avocados keeping the skin intact.

Mash the pulp and add the tuna, shallot, hard boiled egg, mayonnaise, celery and black olives. Season with salt and pepper.

Fill the avocado skins and put them in the refrigerator at least 1 hour before serving.

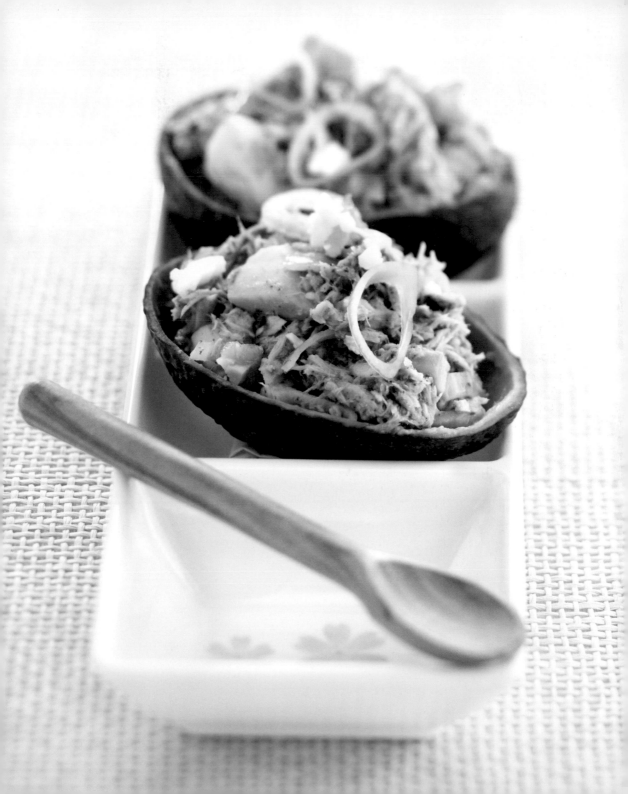

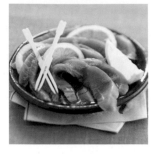

Dill marinated salmon

Serves 4

✴ To do the night before

◼ **Preparation time:**
20 minutes
◼ **Marinating time:**
36 hours

◼ **Ingredients:**
> 1 salmon fillet (around
2¼ lb - 1 kg) with skin
> Juice of ½ lemon
> 3 tablespoons of olive oil
> Salt and pepper

◼ **For the marinade:**
> 4 teaspoons of salt
> 2 tablespoons of fructose
> 2 teaspoons of fresh
ground white pepper
> 1 to 2 large bunches of
chopped dill (8 tablespoons)

Prepare the filet by being careful to remove any bones with a small tweezers.

For the marinade, mix the salt, fructose and pepper. Uniformly divide this dry marinade on the salmon, flesh side only. Knead with your fingers to make it penetrate. Add a thick layer of dill on top.

Tightly wrap with several layers of plastic wrap. Let the salmon marinade for 36 hours in the refrigerator.

Scrape the surface of the salmon to remove the spices, then cut into thin slices.

Prepare a sauce with the lemon juice, olive oil, salt and pepper. Line the individual plates with thin salmon slices, then brush sauce on them. Sprinkle with dill.

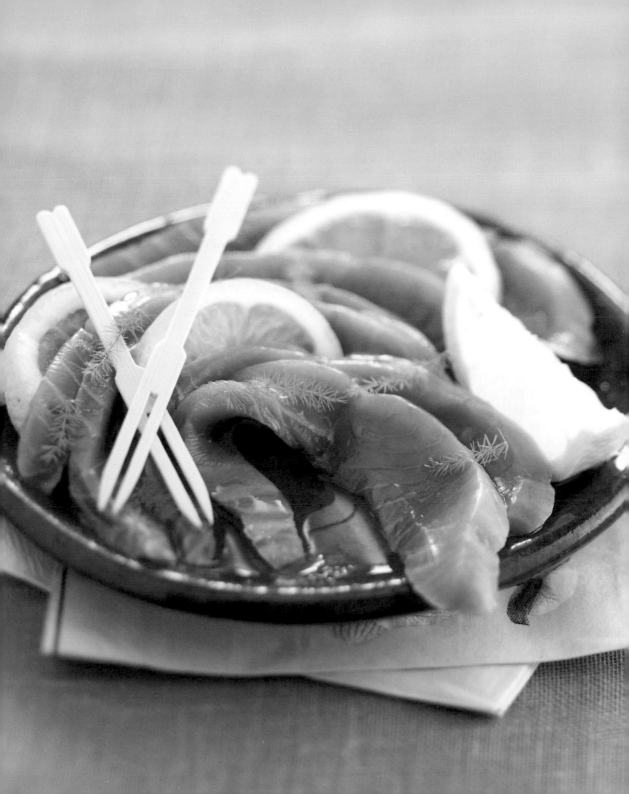

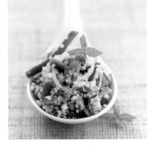

Quinoa à la provençale

Serves 6

■ **Preparation time:**
25 minutes
■ **Cooking time:**
35 minutes

■ **Ingredients:**
> 7oz (200 g) quinoa
> 1 can of extra-thin
green beans (16oz - 450 g)
> 1 peeled tomatoes
in their juice (14oz - 400 g)
> 2 onions
> 3 garlic cloves
> A little olive oil
> 2 teaspoons of tomato
paste
> 7fl oz (20 cl) of fat-free
chicken stock
> 1 pinch of ground
coriander
> 1/2 bunch of fresh mint
> Salt and pepper

Pour the quinoa in a fine strainer. Wash and rinse at length
under cold water. Put two times its volume of water in a pan. Add salt. Bring to a boil and cook covered for 3 minutes. Remove from the flame and let it sit 10 minutes to absorb the water. Set aside.

Drain the green beans well in a strainer. Cut the peeled tomatoes into chucks and let them drain in a strainer.

Peel and chop the onions and garlic. Brown the onions with a little olive oil in a stockpot. Add the garlic then the green beans and the tomato paste, and cook for a few minutes over a high flame stirring constantly.

Sprinkle with the stock and add the tomatoes. Let cook over a low flame from around ten minutes.

Preheat the oven to 180°C. Oil a baking pan. Mix the quinoa and vegetables. Season with salt and pepper and add the coriander. Pour the mixture in the dish, cover with tin foil and put in the oven. Bake 15 to 20 minutes.

Before serving sprinkle the dish with finely chopped fresh mint.

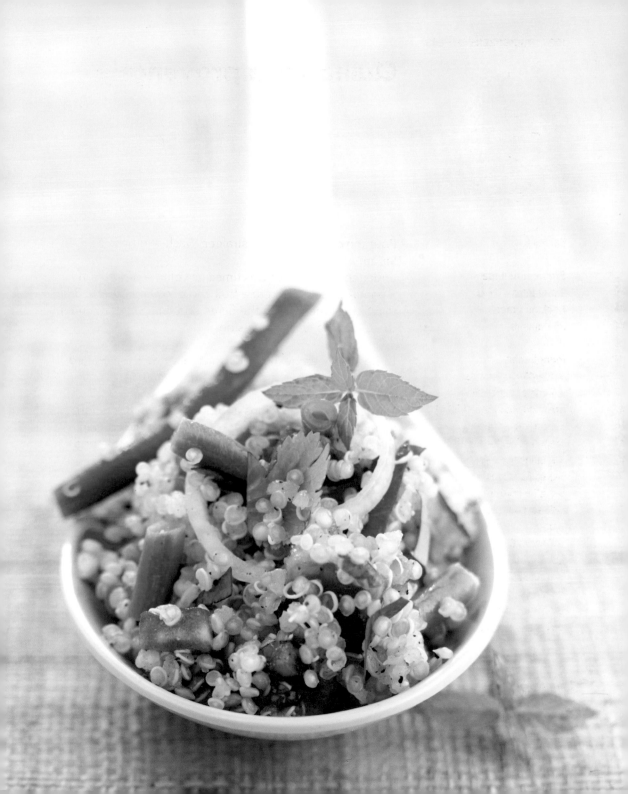

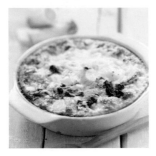

Leek quiche

Serves 6

■ **Preparation time:**
15 minutes
■ **Cooking time:**
1h15 minutes

■ **Ingredients:**
> 1lb (500 g) leeks,
white part
> 7oz (200 g) small bacon
cubes, unsmoked
> 1 large chopped onion
> A little olive oil
> 5 eggs
> 10fl oz (30 cl) low-fat
cream
> A little nutmeg
> 7oz (200 g) grated gruyere
> Salt and pepper

Wash the leeks and cut them into 1 to 2 cm lengths.
Steam them for 20 minutes. Set aside and let drain.

Brown the bacon cubes in a frying pan over a low flame.
Make them let off as much fat as possible. Do not burn
them. Put them on paper towels.

Brown the onion with the olive oil in a frying pan.
Add the drained leeks and stop cooking as soon as they
are tender. Preheat the oven to 160 °C.

Scramble the eggs in a bowl with the cream. Salt very
lightly, pepper and grate a little nutmeg. Add the grated
gruyere. Mix well then add the bacon cubes, onion and
leeks taken from the pan with a skimmer to avoid the
cooking liquid.

Pour the mixture into an oiled baking dish. Bake 40 to
45 minutes. It is preferable, but not necessary, to cook in
a double boiler. Serve warm with a good green or mixed
salad.

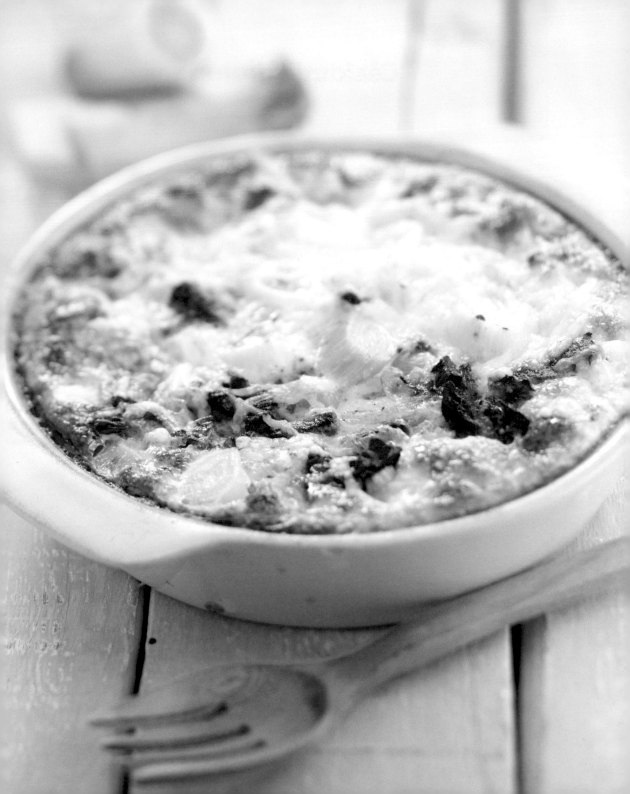

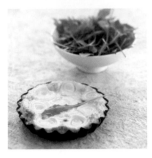

Clafoutis d'oignons

Serves 4

■ **Preparation time:**
15 minutes
■ **Cooking time:**
40 minutes

■ **Ingredients:**
> 10 chopped onions
> A little olive oil
> 4 yolks + 1 egg
> 9fl oz (25 cl) low-fat
liquid cream
> 9oz (250 g) grated gruyere
> Salt and pepper

In a non-stick frying pan, brown the onions over a low flame in the olive oil until they become soft and tender. Do not burn them: stir constantly with a wooden spoon or spatula. Using a skimmer, place the onions on a plate and dry them with paper towels to remove as much oil as possible. Set aside.

Preheat the oven to 170 °C.

In a large bowl beat the yolks and egg, liquid cream and gruyere. Season with salt and pepper. Add the onions. Mix well and pour into an anti-stick pie pan.

Bake 30 to 35 minutes. Unmold and serve hot, warm or cold with a green salad.

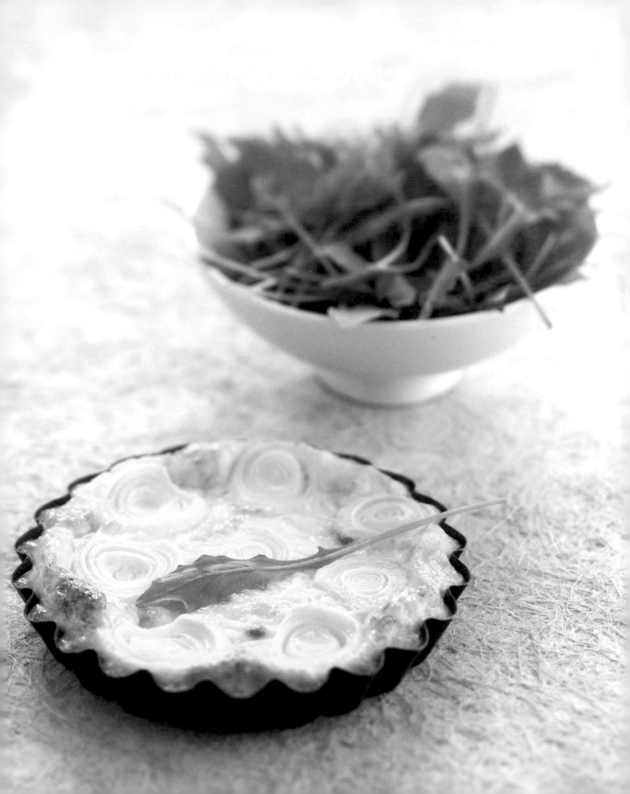

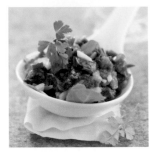

Duck breast tartare

Serves 4

Preparation time:
20 minutes

Refrigeration time:
1 hour

Ingredients:
> 2 shallots
> 3 cornichons
> 10 sprigs of chive
> 2 large duck breasts
(magret), very fresh
> 3 tablespoons of olive oil
> 1/2 teaspoons of fresh
ground black pepper
> 1 tablespoon of
balsamic vinegar
> 1 egg yolk (optional)
> A small watercress salad
> 1 tablespoon of chopped
Italian parsley
> Salt

Peel the shallots and chop finely.

Chop the cornichons and chives finely.

Remove the duck breast skin and all of the fatty layer so you just have the meat. Cut the meat into small pieces.

In a salad bowl mix the olive oil, shallots, cornichons, chives, black pepper, salt, balsamic vinegar and yolk. Whisk. Add the duck breast meat. Mix energetically to coat all the pieces with the vinaigrette. Chill for at least 1 hour.

Mold the individual portions in large ramekins or metallic circles. To serve, unmold in the center of a plate and place watercress around it. Garnish the top with parsley and dress the salad with vinaigrette (olive oil and balsamic vinegar).

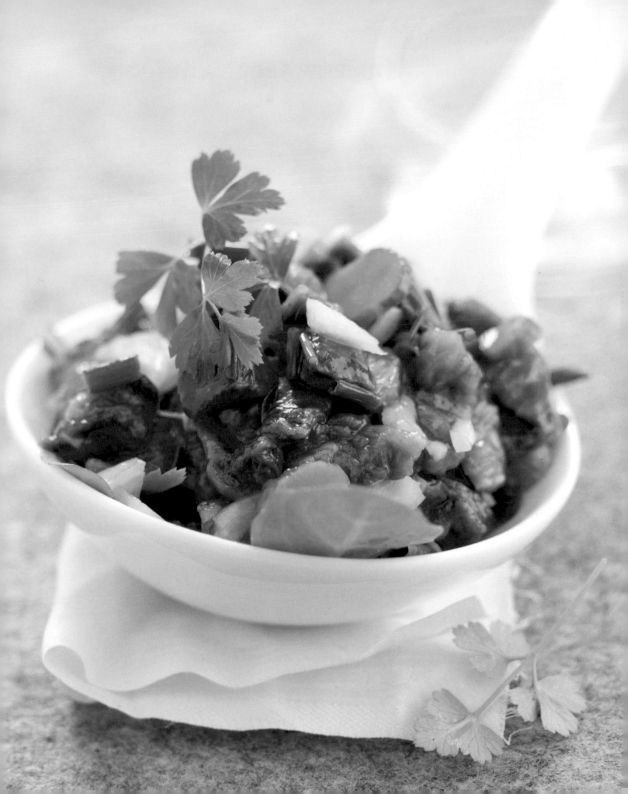

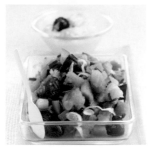

Tuna tartare with aïoli

Serves 4

■ **Preparation time:**
30 minutes

■ **Ingredients:**
> 5 garlic cloves
> 2 egg yolks
> 9fl oz (25 cl) olive oil
> 21oz (600 g) very fresh
tuna filets
> Juice of 3 lemons
> 1 green bell pepper
> 4 shallots
> 1 bunch of chives
> 1 head of lettuce
> 12 cherry tomatoes
> 12 pitted green olives
> Salt and pepper

In a mortar, crush the peeled garlic cloves until obtaining a puree. Add the yolks, a pinch of salt and pepper. Pour the olive oil in a thin stream and whip as if making mayonnaise. Chill the aïoli in a sauceboat.

Drain the tuna, and chop finely with a knife. Sprinkle with lemon juice. Season with salt and pepper and mix. Chill.

Wash the bell pepper, remove the seeds and dice the pulp finely. Chop the shallots and chives finely. Add all of the ingredients to the tuna. Adjust the seasoning.

Make tuna tartare steaks using a ramekin which you unmold with a sharp blow over plates containing a bed of lettuce. Garnish with cherry tomatoes cut in half and olives.

Serve accompanied by the aïoli.

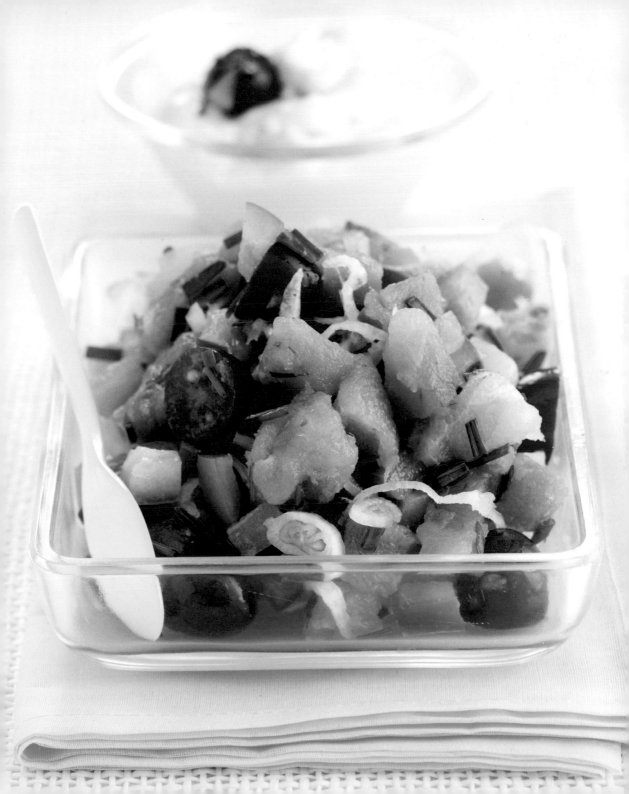

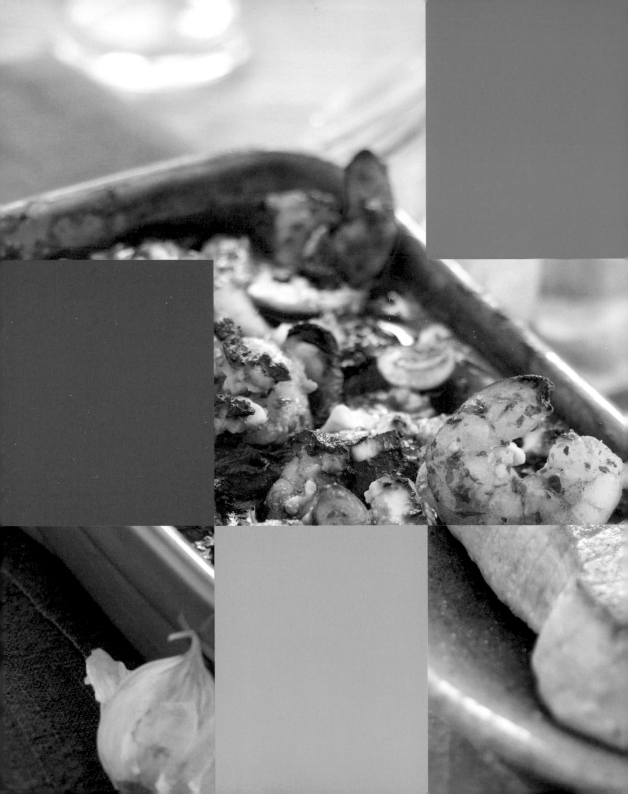

ENTREES

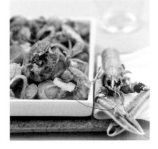

Langoustines with leek fondue

Serves 4

■ **Preparation time:**
30 minutes
■ **Cooking time:**
25 minutes

■ **Ingredients:**
> 5 leeks, white part
> 3 tablespoons of olive oil
> 1 dose of powdered saffron
> 24 uncooked langoustines
> 2fl oz (5 cl) cognac
> 5fl oz (15 cl) low-fat crème fraîche (or soy cream)
> Salt and pepper

Wash the leeks and cut them into thin slices.
Brown them in a frying pan with 1 tablespoon of olive oil.
Cover and cook over a low flame for 15 minutes, stirring regularly. Add the saffron. Season with salt and pepper.

Peel the langoustines using a small scissors. You can leave the tail for a better presentation, but make sure to remove the small black gut.

Sauté the langoustines over a high flame for 3 minutes with 2 tablespoons of olive oil in a frying pan.
At the end of cooking, flambé with cognac.

Place the leeks on a serving platter and put the langoustines on top (you can also use individual plates).

Pour the crème fraîche in the pan where the langoustines were cooked. Put on the burner and deglaze with a spatula. Spread the sauce over the langoustines and serve.

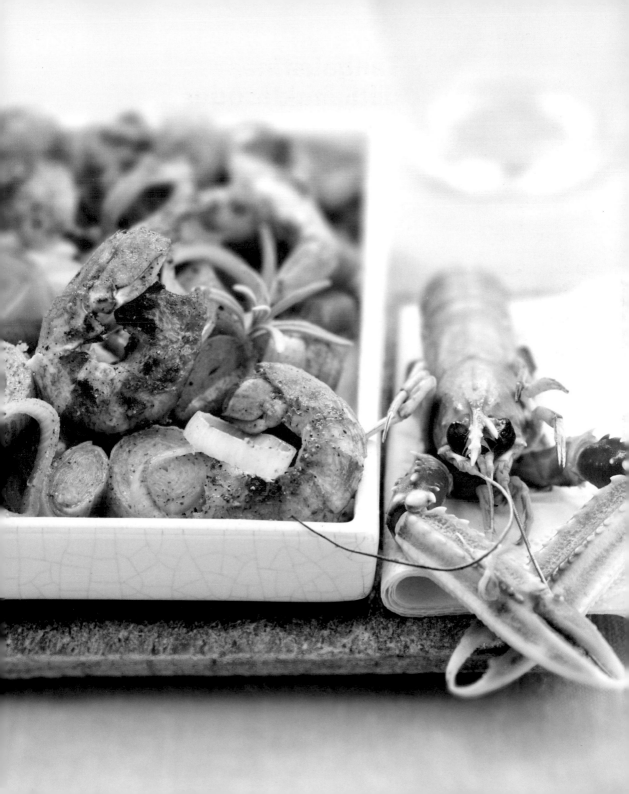

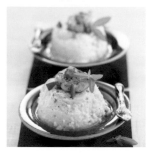

Timbales de Saint-Jacques with prawns

Serves 4

■ **Preparation time:**
10 minutes
■ **Cooking time:**
45 minutes

■ **Ingredients:**
> 8 large scallops
> 8 large whole raw shrimp
> Olive oil
> Ten raw peeled shrimp cut into small pieces
> 1 large egg
> 1 thick whole yogurt
> 1 crushed garlic cloves
> 7fl oz (20 cl) low-fat liquid cream
> 1 bunch Italian parsley
> Salt and pepper

Preheat the oven to 170 °C.

Mix the 8 scallops and have of the shelled prawns with a drizzle of olive oil. Place them in a bowl and add the shrimp, egg, yogurt and garlic. Mix, and season with salt and pepper. Pour into 4 ramekins oiled with olive oil.

Place the ramekins in a baking dish, pour the hot water into the dish and cook for 40 minutes. During this time, shell the remaining prawns. Unmold the ramekins on 4 plates and keep warm.

Five minutes before serving brown the prawn tails in a little olive oil. Season with salt and pepper and set aside.

Deglaze the baking dish with liquid cream.

Place a prawn tail on each timbale, pour the sauce on them and garnish with parsley.

★ This dish can be served with Provencal tomatoes, broccoli, green beans or spinach.

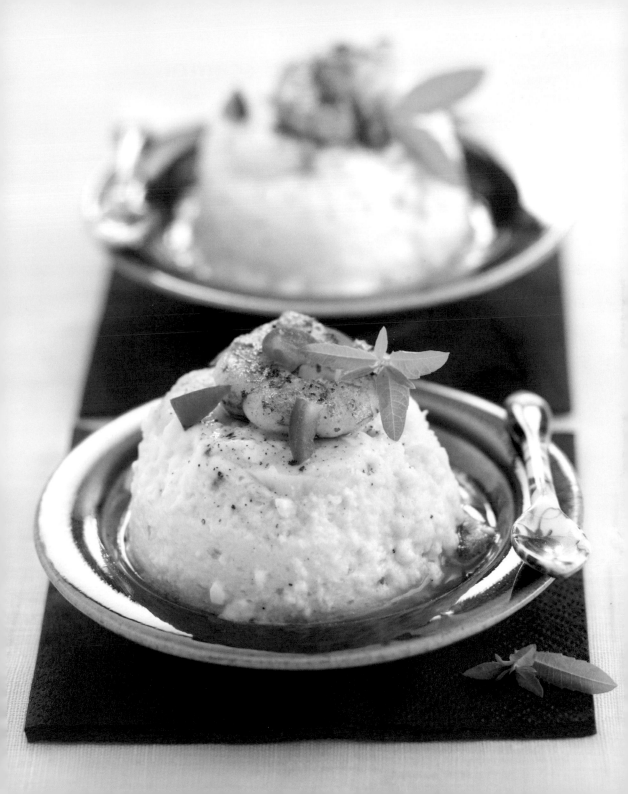

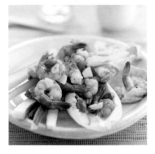

Marinated scampi

Serves 4

■ **Preparation time:**
10 minutes
■ **Refrigeration time:**
1 hour
■ **Cooking time:**
3 minutes

■ **Ingredients:**
> 1¾ to 2¼ lb
(800 g to 1 kg) of raw
scampi (Italian langoustine),
i.e. at least 4 per person
> 9fl oz (25 cl) olive oil
> Juice of 3 lemons
> 3 finely minced garlic
cloves
> 1 bunch chopped parsley
> 4 large tomatoes
> 1 cucumber
> 1 small curly endive
> 1 endive
> Salt and freshly ground
pepper

Poach the scampi in boiling water for 2 minutes, the time it takes them to change color. Put them immediately in cold water to stop the cooking process. Carefully shell them and devein them keeping the tail.

In a bowl whisk the olive oil, lemon juice, garlic and parsley. Season with plenty of salt and pepper. Add the shrimp and make sure they are covered with plenty of marinade. Let them marinade for around 1 hour in the refrigerator.

Drop the tomatoes into boiling water and cook for 40 seconds then rinse under cold water. Peel them and completely empty them only keeping the pulp. Dice them and put them on paper towels.

Cut the cucumber lengthwise into quarters. Remove the seeds and keep the flesh. Recut each piece into two to obtain 8 strips.

On each plate, put the cucumber strips around the edge, make a bed with the curly endive leaves and arrange 3 endive leafs in a star. Remove the shrimp from the marinade, cut them in half lengthwise and arrange them on the salad so that they form a crown. Pour the marinade over them and garnish with the diced tomatoes.

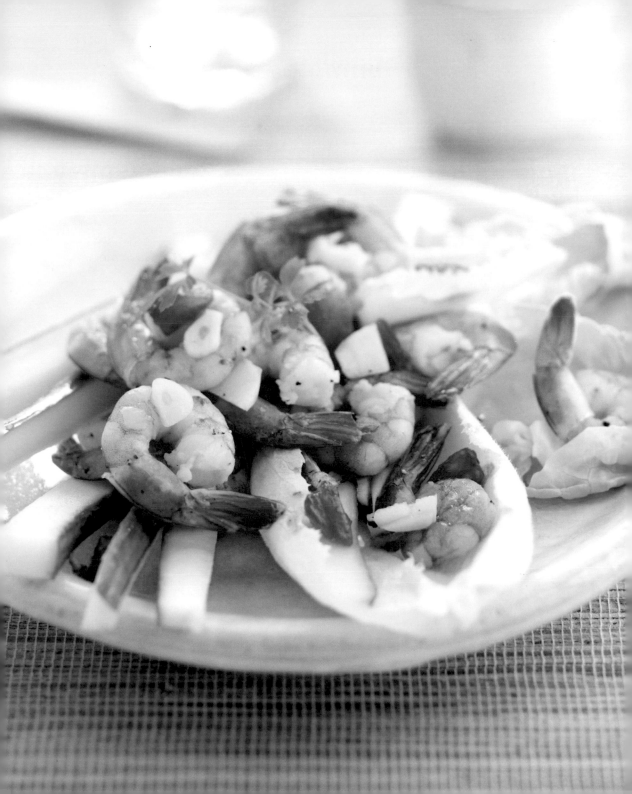

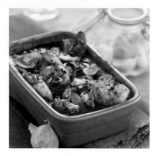

Shrimp gratin

Serves 4

■ **Preparation time:**
40 minutes
■ **Cooking time:**
30 minutes

■ **Ingredients:**
> 2¼ lb (1 kg) of medium
raw shrimp
> Juice of 1 lemon
> 4 ripe tomatoes
> 3 spring onions
> 3 garlic cloves
> 3 tablespoons of olive oil
> 4fl oz (10 cl) dry
white wine
> 5oz (150 g) feta cheese
> 1 tablespoon of finely
chopped dill
> Salt and pepper

Shell shrimp and keep the tails. Rinse them then leave them in a strainer. Season with salt and pepper and sprinkle with lemon juice. Set aside.

Boil the tomatoes for 40 seconds. Cool them in cold water and then peel them and remove the seeds. Dice the flesh.

Eliminate the roots and stalk ends from the onions. Wash and chop them. Cut the garlic cloves into thin slices.

Heat the olive oil in a frying pan. Sauté the shrimp 1 to 2 minutes stirring well so that they are cooked on all surfaces. Remove them and set aside.

In the same oil lightly brown the onion and garlic for 1 to 2 minutes. Add the tomatoes then the white wine. Let the sauce simmer 10 to 15 minutes uncovered over a low flame. Preheat the oven to 220 °C.

Divide the shrimp on four individual ovenproof dishes (or one large one). Coat with tomato sauce and then crumble the feta on top. Place in oven and let the cheese melt from 10 to 12 minutes.

Sprinkle with dill before serving.

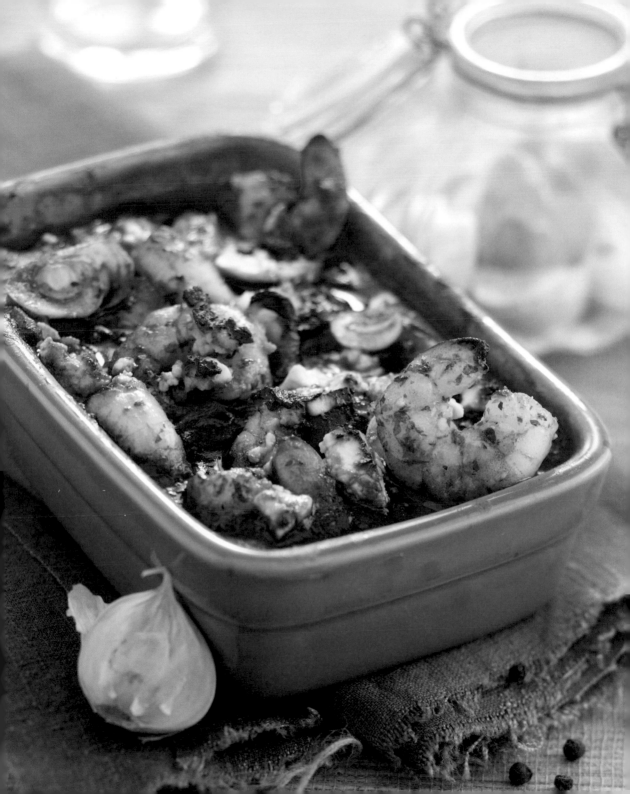

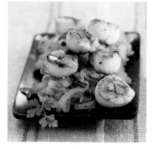

Poêlée
de Saint-Jacques
(scallops) aux échalotes

Serves 4

■ **Preparation time:**
10 minutes
■ **Cooking time:**
10 minutes

■ **Ingredients:**
> 20 shallots
> 2 tablespoons of olive oil
> A knob of goose fat
> 16 cleaned scallops
> 2 sprigs Italian parsley
> Salt and pepper

Peel the shallots and roughly chop them widthwise. Brown them over a low flame in the olive oil, avoid burning them. Constantly stir with a spatula, lightly season with sale and pepper. Put them on paper towels to remove the oil. Keep warm.

Melt the goose fat in a frying pan. Dry the scallops, then sear them over a high flame for around 1 minute on each side. Season with salt and pepper.

Garnish each plate with a bed of shallots, place the scallops and garnish with parsley.

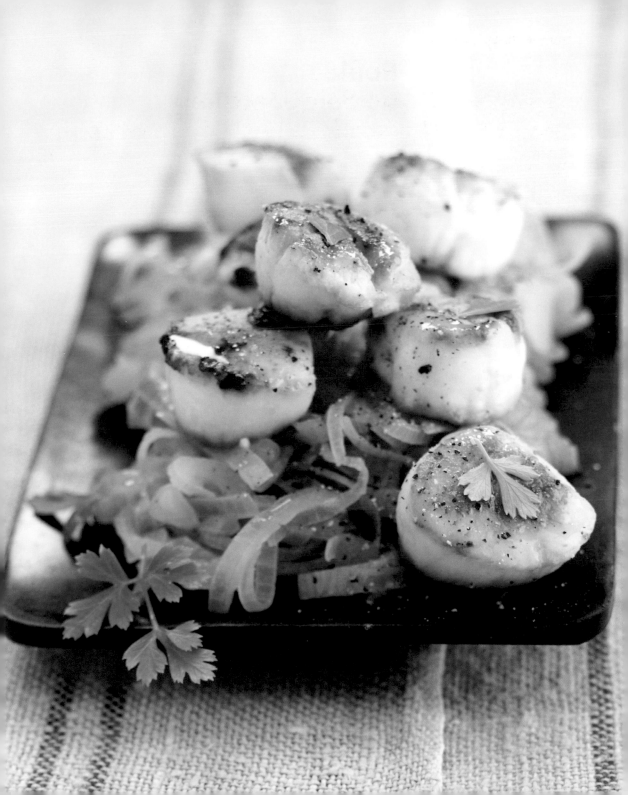

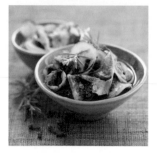

Squid
à la provençale

Serves 4

■ **Preparation time:**
25 minutes
■ **Cooking time:**
40 minutes

■ **Ingredients:**
>2¼ lb (1 kg) of pf small
prepared squid
> 4 onions
> 5 garlic cloves
> 4 tablespoons of olive oil
> 14fl oz (40 cl) dry
white wine
> 1 jar of tomato paste
(5oz - 150 g)
> 1 clove
> 3 large pinches of nutmeg
> 1 sprig of thyme
> 1 bay leaf
> 1 sprig of rosemary
> 2 or 3 pinches of cinnamon
> Salt and pepper

Wash the squid, drain them and cut them in slices.
Cut the tentacles at the level of the eyes.

Peel the onions and chop them. Peel and chop the garlic.
Heat the olive oil in a frying pan and let the onions
soften not letting them turn black.

Add the garlic and pieces of squid. Let them release a
little water for 2 to 3 minutes cooking over a high flame,
stirring with a spatula. Lower the flame. Add the white
wine, tomato paste, clove and nutmeg. Season with salt
and pepper and mix. Add the thyme, bay leaf, rosemary
and cinnamon. Bring to a boil and then lower the flame.
Cover and let simmer for 15 minutes. Remove the cover,
stir and let the sauce reduce further for around 10 minutes. Remove the thyme, rosemary and bay leaf.
Adjust the seasoning.

Serve warm in individual terra cotta dishes.

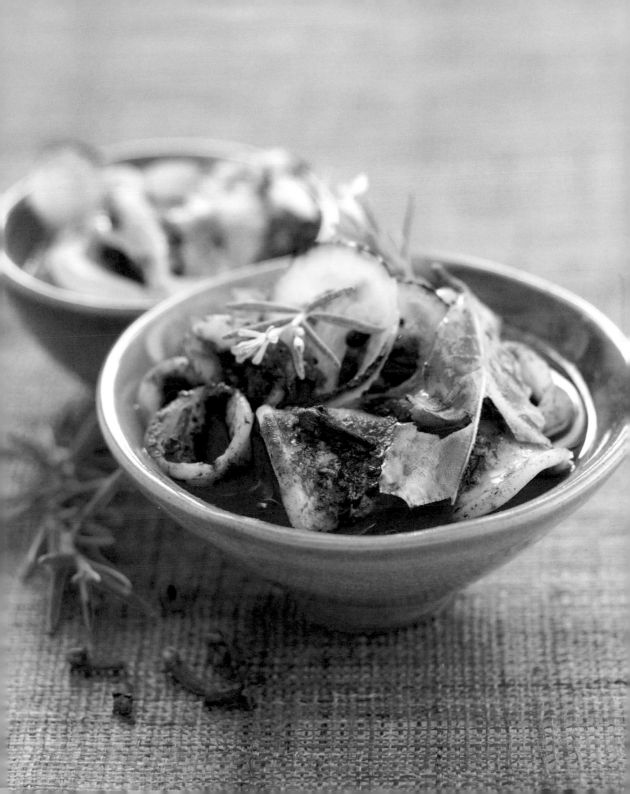

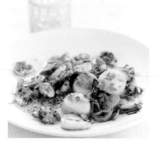

Saint-Jacques (scallops) aux champignons

Serves 4

■ **Preparation time:**
20 minutes
■ **Cooking time:**
35 minutes

■ **Ingredients:**
> 2 tablespoons of
wine vinegar
> 3 shallots
> 1 small bunch of parsley
> 1 tablespoon of herbes
de Provence
> 12 scallops
> 1lb (500 g) of champi-
gnons
> 3 tablespoons of olive oil
> 9fl oz (25 cl) low-fat liquid
crème fraîche
> Salt and pepper

Prepare a court-bouillon with 250 ml of water, vinegar, shallots cut into slices, a little chopped parsley and herbes de Provence. Season with salt and pepper. Let the court-bouillon simmer on a low flame for 10 minutes.

Prepare the scallops by separating the meat from the coral. Eliminate the black parts and the nerves. Put them in the court-bouillon. Let them poach 2 minutes on a very low flame. Drain and keep the meat and coral set aside separately.

Remove the dirty end from the champignons. Wash them, dry them on paper towels and peel them. Cut into thin slices.

In a frying pan, heat the olive oil and slightly brown the champignons regularly stirring with a spatula. Season with salt and pepper.

Add the scallops and the crème fraîche. Let them cook over a low flame for 2 minutes. Then add the coral. Let cook for another 2 or 3 minutes, just to reduce the sauce. Attention, the scallops need to remain very tender. If they are cooked too much they become rubbery.

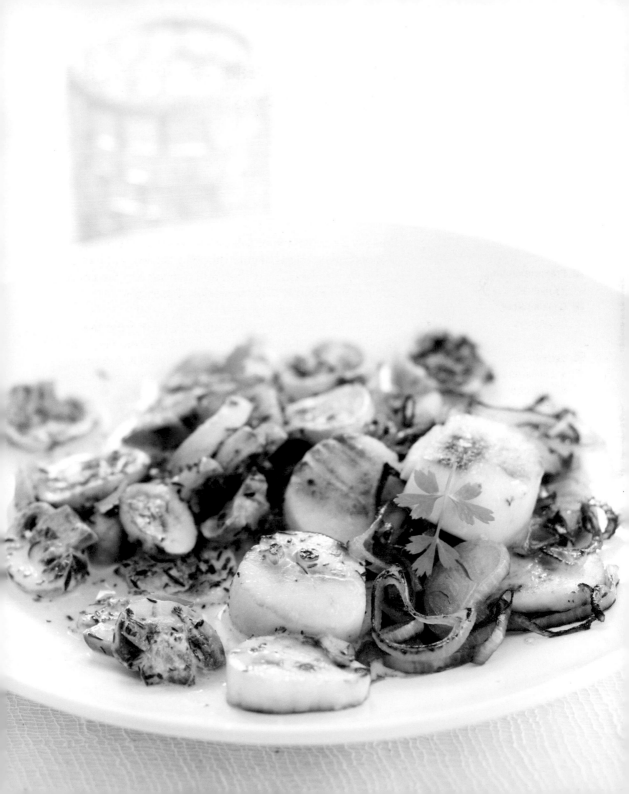

Zucchini stuffed with crab

Serves 4

■ **Preparation time:**
30 minutes
■ **Cooking time:**
35 minutes

■ **Ingredients:**
> 2 or 3 large zucchini
> 1 can of peeled
tomatoes (9oz - 250 g)
> 5oz (150 g) canned crab
> 3 onions
> Olive oil
> 1 bunch of parsley
> 2 tablespoons of
grated parmesan
> Salt and pepper

Wash and dry the zucchini. Blanche them 5 to 6 minutes in boiling water. Let them drain and cool.

Preheat the oven to 220 °C. During that time, drain the tomatoes and crumble the crab. Peel the onions and chop them. Brown them with the olive oil in a frying pan.

Cut the tomatoes into pieces and drain them. Add them to the onions and cook for 5-6 minutes stirring. Chop the parsley and add to the mixture. Season with salt and pepper. Off the flame, add the crumbled crab.

Cut the zucchini in half lengthwise. Empty them with a spoon so that their thickness is less than 1 cm.
Chop the obtained flesh and add it to the mixture.

Put the zucchini on an oiled baking dish, and fill them with the stuffing. Sprinkle with parmesan and drizzle with some olive oil. Bake 15 to 20 minutes.

Bouillabaisse de l'Atlantique

Serves 6

■ **Preparation time:**
30 minutes
■ **Cooking time:**
1h30 minutes

■ **Ingredients:**
> 2 large chopped onions
> 6 tablespoons of olive oil
> 2 minced garlic cloves
> 1 bouquet garni
> 18fl oz (50 cl) dry
white wine
> 1 large tomato
> 1 teaspoon of mild paprika
> 1/2 teaspoon of
Cayenne pepper
> Hake head
> 21oz (600 g) conger
> 21oz (600 g) monkfish filet
> 8 langoustines
> 1 liter of mussels
> Chopped parsley
> Salt and pepper

Sauté the onions with 2 tablespoons of olive oil in a frying pan. Halfway through the cooking add the garlic and bouquet garni. Pour in the white wine, add the tomato cut in quarters, the paprika and pepper and hake head. Let it reduce by half. Add 1 liter of water and cook over a low flame for 45 minutes. Let it cool 15 minutes and put through a conical strainer.

Cut the conger and monkfish. Sauté the pieces of fish in 4 tablespoons of olive oil in a large pot, season with salt and pepper. Add the langoustines and pour in the bouillon. Heat just to the boiling point, add the mussels, let it heat until boiling for a few minutes until the mussels are open. Adjust the seasoning.

Serve in large soup plates (or bowls) and sprinkle with chopped parsley.

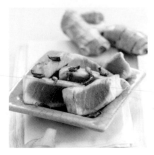

Tuna filet with ginger

Serves 4

■ **Preparation time:**
10 minutes
■ **Cooking time:**
10 minutes
■ **Marinating time:**
1 hour

■ **Ingredients:**
> 2oz (50 g) of fresh ginger
> 4 tablespoons of tamari
> 4 tablespoons of olive oil
> Juice of 1 lemon
> 21oz (600 g) very fresh
tuna fillet – 3 cm thick
> 2 sprigs Italian parsley
> Pepper

Peel the ginger and chop very finely with a knife.

In a bowl prepare the marinade with the tamari, olive oil, lemon juice and ginger. Season with pepper. Let the tuna filet marinate at least 1 hour at room temperature. Turn the fish every now and then. Preheat the oven to 100 °C.

Pour the marinade into a pan and heat over a high flame. Sear the tuna 1 minute on each side spraying the top of the filet with the boiling marinade. The tuna needs to stay raw inside.

On a chopping board, cut the filet into wide slices 2 to 3 cm each. Place them on a plate and keep warm in the oven.

During this time, reduce the marinade over a low flame. When it starts to get a little thicker, spread it uniformly over the tuna. Leave it in the oven for another 2 minutes. Before serving, garnish with a few leaves of Italian parsley.

★ This dish can be served with steamed broccoli, snow peas (see pg. 216) or Montignac ratatouille (see pg. 212).

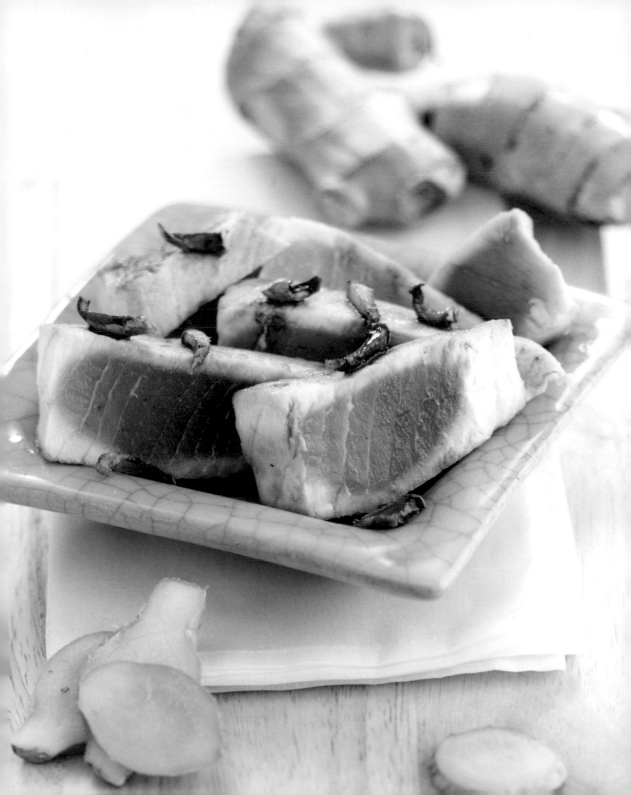

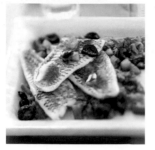

Red mullet
with anchoïade

Serves 4

■ **Preparation time:**
15 minutes
■ **Cooking time:**
15 minutes

■ **Ingredients:**
> 1 can of anchovy fillets
in olive oil
> 2 teaspoons of
balsamic vinegar
> 5 fresh tomatoes
> 12 black olives
> 3 dried tomatoes
> 1 red bell pepper
> 3 tablespoons of
olive oil
> 8 red mullet filets
> Salt and pepper

Prepare the anchoïade by mixing the anchovy filets, balsamic vinegar and a part of the oil from the can of anchovies. Set aside.

Boil the tomatoes for 40 seconds then rinse under cold water. Peel and deseed them. Dice the flesh into small pieces and put them on paper towels. Pit the black olives. Coarsely chop them and then the dry tomatoes. Cut the bell pepper in half, deseed it and then cut into small cubes.

In a preheated frying pan, pour the olive oil and then sauté the chopped bell pepper then the fresh tomatoes. During the last minute of cooking, add the olives and the dried tomatoes. Season with salt and pepper. Keep warm.

Grill the red mullet filets on both sides, either under the broiler or in a non-stick pan with a little olive oil.

Divide a side dish you've selected on four individual plates. Put the red mullet filets on top, the tomato mixture and pour a little of the anchoïade on top and around the plate as decoration.

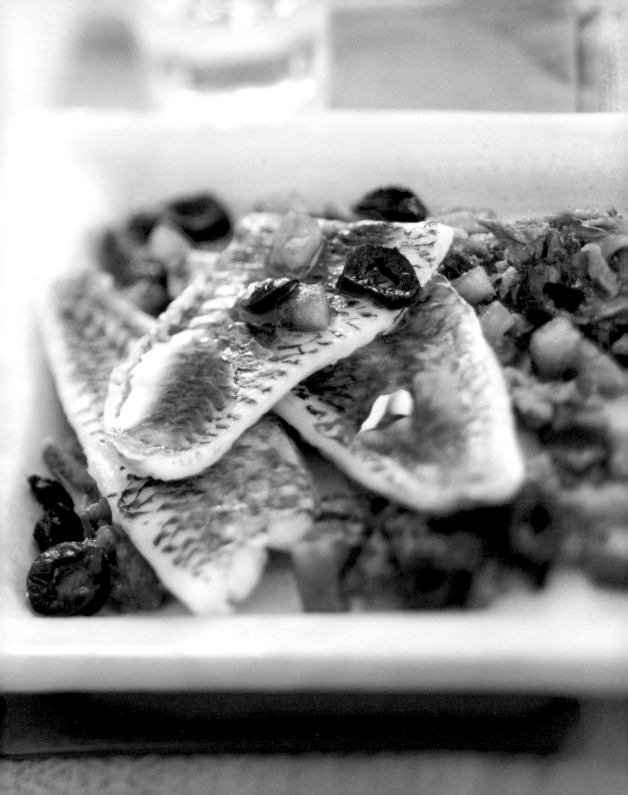

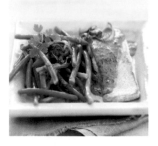

Salmon filet with olive cream

Serves 4

■ **Preparation time:**
10 minutes
■ **Cooking time:**
20 minutes

■ **Ingredients:**
> 3 tablespoons of olive oil
> 4 fresh salmon filets
(around 7oz or 200 g)
with skin
> 7oz (200 g) black olives
> 3 chopped shallots
> 5fl oz (15 cl) soy cream
(or low-fat whipping cream)
> Salt and pepper

In a non-stick pan, pout two tablespoons of olive oil, and cook the salmon filets for twelve minutes on the skin side over a low flame. At the last minute, turn the filets and sear them one minute on the top.

Pit the black olives and puree them. Keep a couple of olives cut into slices for garnishing.

Sauté the shallots with 1 tablespoon of olive oil in a frying pan. Lightly season with salt. Reduce by two thirds, then add the olive puree. Let it cook for 1 minute while stirring. Off the flame, add the soy cream. Adjust the seasoning.

Remove the skin from the filets with a thin knife.

Arrange the filets on individual plates. Pour the sauce over them. Garnish with the remaining olives and arrange the vegetable side dish around them.

✷ This dish can be served with steamed broccoli, snow peas (see pg. 216) or Montignac ratatouille (see pg. 212).

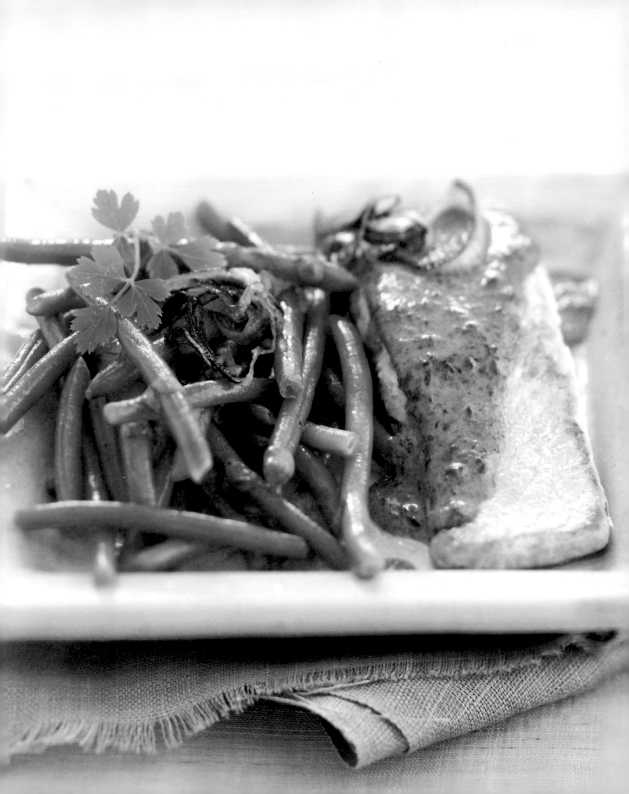

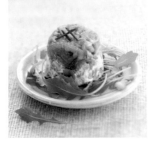

Salmon tartare
with fresh goat cheese

Serves 4

■ **Preparation time:**
25 minutes
■ **Marinating time:**
30 minutes
■ **Refrigeration time:**
2 hours

■ **Ingredients:**
> 7 to 8 tablespoons
of olive oil
> Juice of 2 lemons
> 1/2 bunch of dill
> 1/2 bunch of chives
> 21oz (600 g) salmon filet
> 7oz (200 g) of fresh goat
cheese
> 14oz (400 g) arugula
> Salt and pepper

Mix the 5 tablespoons of olive oil, the lemon juice, half
the dill and half the chopped chives. Season with salt
and pepper.

Cut the salmon into pieces and put it in the marinade
for at least 30 minutes. Remove the salmon and keep
the marinade. Coarsely chop the salmon to make the
tartare.

Soften the goat cheese by mixing it with a fork with 1
tablespoon of olive oil. Season with pepper. Add the
marinade and whisk until obtaining a thick cream.
Add the salmon tartare. Stir energetically to obtain a
uniform mixture.

Fill oiled circles or ramekins. Cover them with plastic
wrap and leave in the refrigerator for around 2 hours.

When serving, place the arugula on individual plates.
Unmold the ramekins with a sharp blow onto the center
of the plate, add the herbs set aside for the decoration
and possibly a little vinaigrette on the side of the plate.

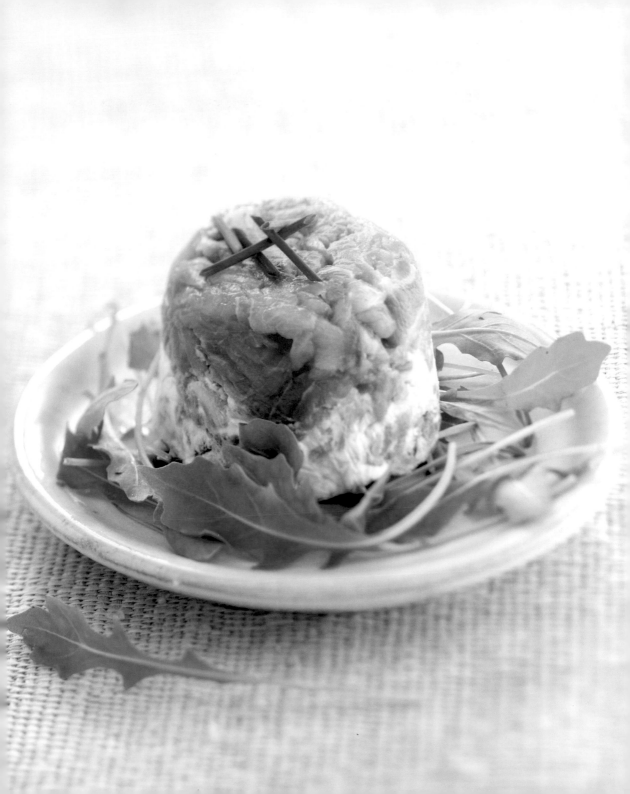

Dorade à l'andalouse

Serves 4

■ **Preparation time:**
15 minutes
■ **Cooking time:**
25 to 40 minutes

■ **Ingredients:**
> 4 small sea breams 21oz
(600 g) each or one sea
bream 5½ lb (2.5 kg)
> 7fl oz (20 cl) +2 table-
spoons of olive oil
> 2 tablespoons
of garlic powder
> 4 tablespoons of
herbes de Provence
> A dozen garlic cloves
> 2 lemons
> Salt and pepper

Preheat the oven to 200 °C. Put the sea bream/s in a large baking dish. Sprinkle a little olive oil. Season with salt and pepper. Sprinkle the garlic powder and herbes de Provence. Bake for 25 minutes for the small sea bream and 40 minutes for a large one.

During this time cut the garlic cloves into thin slices 1 mm thick. Pour 7fl oz (20 cl) olive oil in a pan. Season with salt and pepper and add the sliced garlic. Cook over a medium flame until the garlic is slightly browned. Do not burn it. Set aside.

Take the sea bream out of the oven. Open it carefully removing the central bone and then arrange it opened up on a warm serving platter.
When serving, put the pan with garlic and oil back on the flame. Pour the boiling oil over the fish filets, uni-formly dividing the garlic bits. Each diner can then add lemon juice as desired.

Monkfish with champignons and red wine

Serves 4

■ **Preparation time:**
20 minutes
■ **Cooking time:**
25 minutes

■ **Ingredients:**
> 14oz (400 g) of
champignons
> 5 shallots
> 3 tablespoons of goose fat
> 9fl oz (25 cl) of
very tanniny red wine
(côtes-du-rhône)
> 1 tablespoon of finely
chopped tarragon
> 2¼ lb (1 kg) monkfish
> 1 bunch of chervil
> Salt and pepper

Cut of the sandy part of the champignons before washing them. Chop them with a big knife. Peel the shallots and chop them very finely.

In a large pan, melt 2 tablespoons of goose fat. Sauté the shallots. Add the champignons. Mix well and sauté the mixture, constantly stirring, until all of the natural moisture of the champignons disappears.

Pour in the red wine and let it reduce by half over a medium flame. Add the tarragon to the sauce and let it reduce further over a low flame until obtaining a type of puree. Season with salt and pepper. Keep warm.

Rinse the monkfish and remove the pieces of remaining skin. Dry it with paper towels and cut it into 3 to 4 cm thick slices. Season with salt and pepper on all sides. Heat 1 tablespoon of goose fat in a non-stick pan. Sear the fish 3 to 4 minutes on each side.

During this time, rinse the chervil. Keep a few sprigs for garnish. Chop the rest and add it to the champignon puree.

Arrange the pieces of fish on warm individual plates. Surround it with champignon puree and garnish with the remaining chervil sprigs.

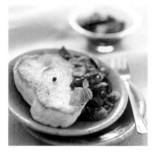

Tuna filet with tomato

Serves 4

■ **Preparation time:**
15 minutes

■ **Cooking time:**
15 minutes

■ **Ingredients:**
> 2¼ lb (1 kg) of ripe
tomatoes
> 3 onions
> 4 tablespoons of olive oil
> 1 tablespoon of
tomato paste
> 4fl oz (10 cl) white wine
> 1/2 teaspoon of
ground ginger
> 1 pinch of saffron
> 2 pinches of
Cayenne pepper
> 5oz (150 g) chopped
black olives
> 4 cuts of tuna filet
> A few basil leaves

Boil the tomatoes for 40 seconds then rinse under cold water. Peel them, cut into quarters and deseed. Cut the flesh into small chucks and let them drain in a strainer.

Peel the onions and chop them. Sauté them in a pan with 2 tablespoons of olive oil until they are soft, do not burn them. Add the tomatoes, tomato paste and white wine. Add the ginger, saffron, Cayenne pepper and chopped olives. Cook over a low flame, stirring to eva-porate as much liquid as possible. This way you'll obtain a thicker sauce. Set aside.

Dry the fish with paper towels. In a very hot frying pan containing 2 tablespoons of olive oil, sear the tuna filets 1 minute per side, then again for 30 seconds.

Arrange the tuna on a platter, or by portions on indivi-dual plates. Coat with the sauce and garnish with a few basil leaves. Drizzle with fresh olive oil.

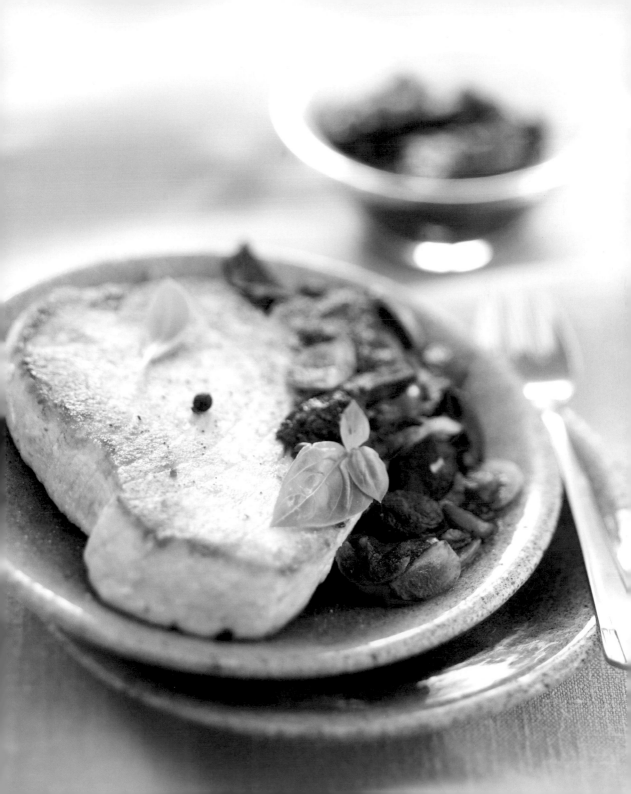

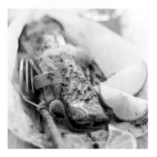

Salmon filets in foil parcels

Serves 4

■ **Preparation time:**
20 minutes
■ **Cooking time:**
15 minutes

■ **Ingredients:**
> 4 leeks, white part
> 4 shallots
> Olive oil
> 4 salmon filets
> 4 sprigs of dill
> Juice of 2 limes
> Salt

Wash and peel the leeks. Cut into lengths around 5 cm long. Cut into slices and then julienne. Peel the shallots and chop them.

Heat 1 tablespoon of olive oil in a pan. Sauté the shallots. Add the julienne leeks. Mix. Cover and let soften over a medium flame for 3 minutes. Uncover, stir and leave over the flame for 1 or 2 minutes. Set aside. Preheat the oven to 220°C.

Cut 4 rectangles out of greaseproof paper or aluminum foil. Remove the skin from the salmon filets. Dry them on paper towels and salt on both sides.

Chop the dill. Mix the dill with the leeks. Divide half the vegetables on the open paper, then place the salmon filets. Sprinkle each filet with lemon juice. Cover with the rest of the vegetables.

Close the paper by putting one of the long ends over the other. Bend the ends well to ensure a good seal. Bake for 10 minutes.

Open the paper and sprinkle with lemon juice and drizzle with olive oil.

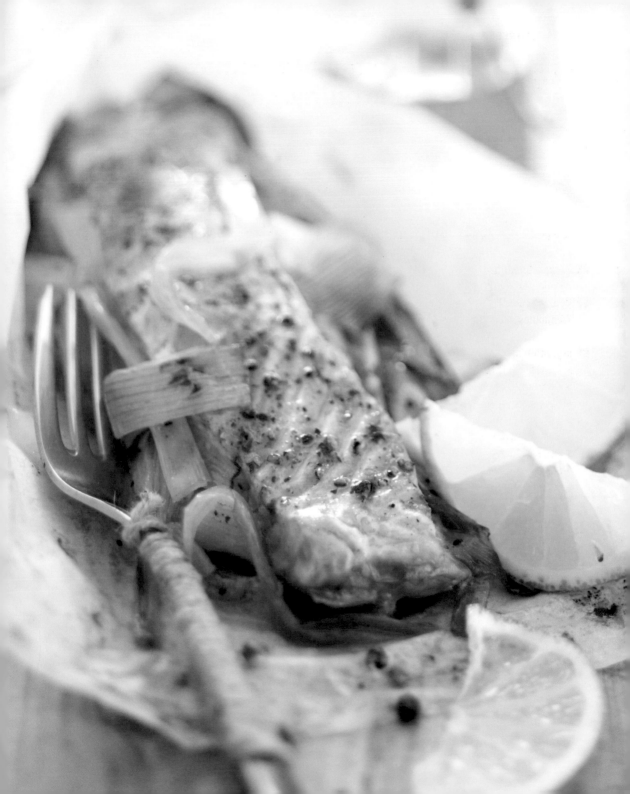

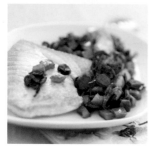

Tuna with tomato and olives

Serves 4

■ **Preparation time:**
25 minutes

■ **Cooking time:**
30 minutes

■ **Ingredients:**
> 1lb (500 g) tomatoes
> 3½ oz (100 g) pitted
black olives
> 1 green bell pepper
in cubes
> 3 garlic cloves
> 4 shallots
> 4 tablespoons of olive oil
> 4fl oz (10 cl) red wine
> 1 bunch of oregano
> 4 slices of tuna filet 5oz
(150 g)
> Juice of 1 lemon
> 3 sprigs Italian parsley
> Salt and pepper

Drop the tomatoes into boiling water and cook for 40 seconds then rinse under cold water. Peel them, deseed and cut the flesh into chunks. Chop half of the olives.

Peel the garlic and shallots and chop them finely. Heat 2 tablespoons of olive oil in a pan and sauté the bell pepper, garlic and shallots. Pour in the red wine and deglaze with a wood spatula. Add the tomatoes and stir. Season with salt and pepper. Cover and let simmer for 5 minutes over a low flame.

Add the chopped black olives and let reduce into a puree uncovered for a few minutes. Add the oregano leaves and then the rest of the olives. Preheat the oven to 210 °C.

Dry the tuna with paper towels. Sprinkle them with lemon juice. Let sit for 2 minutes. Season with salt and pepper.

Heat 2 tablespoons of olive oil in a frying pan.
When it is very hot, brown the tuna 1 minute on each side.

Place the tuna in a baking dish. Coat with the sauce and let it bake for 10 minutes. Before serving, sprinkle with the Italian parsley.

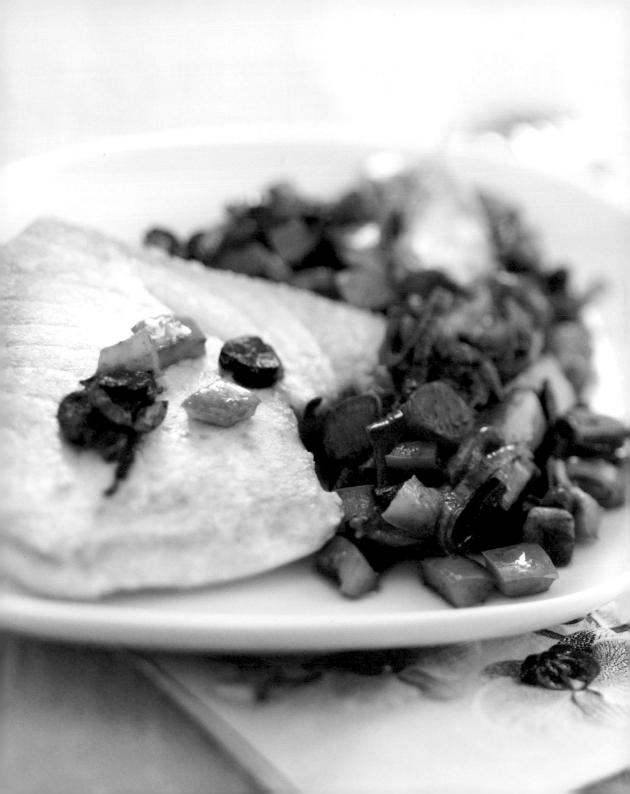

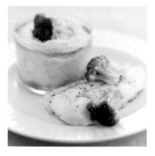

Cod with broccoli

Serves 4

■ **Preparation time:**
25 minutes
■ **Cooking time:**
45 minutes

■ **Ingredients:**
> 28oz (800 g) broccoli
> 3 shallots
> 5 tablespoons of olive oil
> 4 sprigs Italian parsley
> 5fl oz (15 cl) low-fat
crème fraîche
> 4 eggs
> 2 pinches of grated nutmeg
> 5fl oz (15 cl) of
vegetable stock
> 5fl oz (15 cl) white wine
> 1 tablespoon of
chopped thyme
> 4 cod filets (around 7oz
- 200 g) with skin
> Salt and pepper

Divide the broccoli into small bunches, remove the stems and chop coarsely.

Peel the shallots. Chop them and soften them with 2 tablespoons of olive oil. Keep 11oz (300 g) of the broccoli as garnish, add the rest to the shallots. Let cook over a low flame for ten minutes while stirring. Chop the parsley (keep a little for garnish) and add it to the broccoli. Preheat the oven to 210 °C.

Oil 4 ramekins. Puree the broccoli. Add the cream and beaten eggs. Season with salt and pepper and nutmeg. Pour it in the ramekins and then place them in a deep baking pan. Add hot water to the pan and bake for around 25 minutes.

Pour the stock and wine into a pan. Bring to a boil. Add the thyme. Add the broccoli put aside for garnish. Cook for 5 minutes.

Dry the fish with paper towels. Season the flesh side with salt and pepper. Cook it in a pan in 3 tablespoons of olive oil, 5 minutes on the skin side and only 2 minutes on the flesh side.

Unmold the flans on the plates with a sharp blow. Arrange the fish, flesh side up, surrounded by broccoli. Drizzle with olive oil and garnish with parsley.

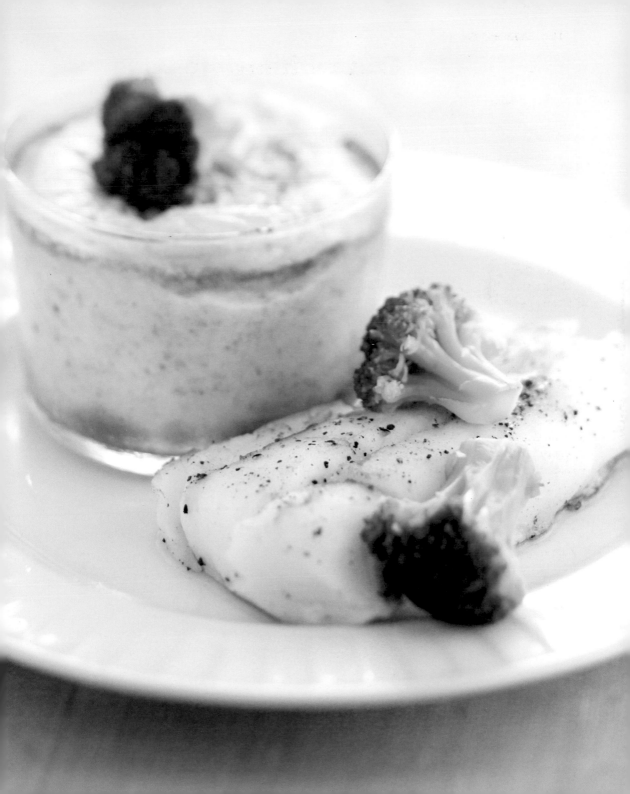

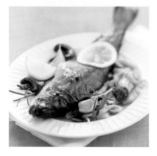

Trout with white wine

Serves 4

■ **Preparation time:**
25 minutes
■ **Cooking time:**
35 minutes

■ **Ingredients:**
> 4 cleaned trout, at least 9oz
(250 g) each
> 4 sprigs of fresh rosemary
> 11oz (300 g) of
champignons
> 2 untreated lemons
> 3 garlic cloves
> 2 leeks
> 2 tablespoons of olive oil
> 7fl oz (20 cl) dry
white wine
> Salt and pepper

Season the inside and outside of the trout with salt and pepper. Place a sprig of rosemary in each fish.

Cut off the sandy part of the champignons before washing them. Chop them.

Cut on lemon into thin slices. Remove the zest from the other lemon and squeeze the juice. Chop the garlic cloves.

Wash the leeks and only keep the edible part. Cut them into thin slices. Preheat the oven to 210 °C.

Put the olive oil into the bottom of a baking pan. Arrange the champignons and 4 trout, then cover them with the leeks and lemon slices. Arrange the lemon zest on top. Mix the white wine, lemon juice and garlic then moisten the contents of the pan. Make a cover with a large sheet of foil and seal the pan. Bake for 35 minutes.

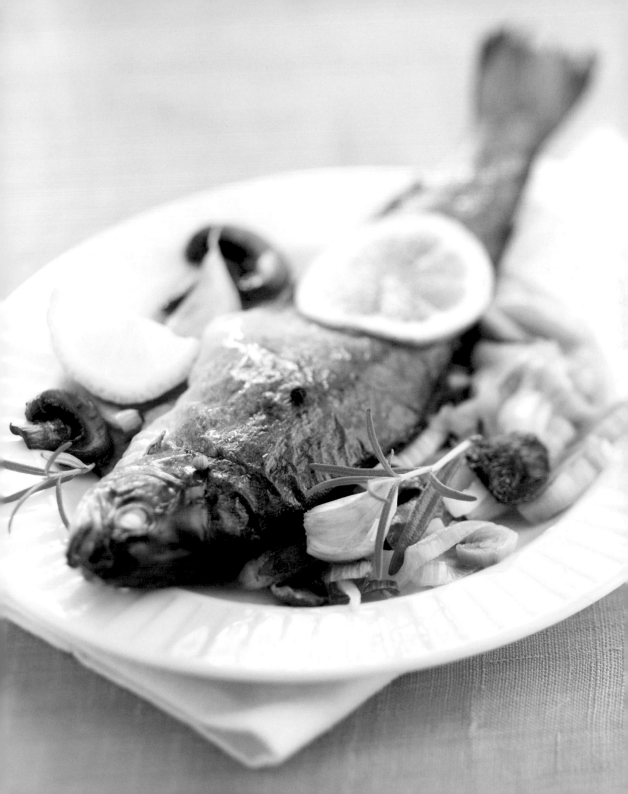

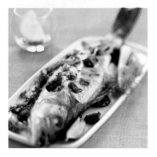

Sea bass with fennel

Serves 4

■ **Preparation time:**
20 minutes

■ **Cooking time:**
50 minutes

■ **Ingredients:**
> 3 large tomatoes
> 2 shallots
> 3 garlic cloves
> 3 tablespoons of olive oil
> 5fl oz (15 cl) white wine
> 1 teaspoon of fennel seeds
> 4 fennel stalks
> 1 large sea bass (cleaned) at least 3¼ lb (1.5 kg) or 2 of 1¾ lb (800 g)
> Salt and pepper

Drop the tomatoes into boiling water and cook for 40 seconds then rinse under cold water. Peel them, deseed and cut the flesh into chunks.

Peel and chop the shallots and garlic. Chop them and soften them with 2 tablespoons of olive oil in a frying pan. Add the chopped tomato and let it reduce for a few minutes. Pour in the white wine. Season with the fennel seeds, salt and pepper. Let simmer over a low flame for 10 to 15 minutes. Preheat the oven to 200 °C.

Fold the two fennel stalks in half and slide them into the fish. Season with salt and pepper. Coat the bass with 1 tablespoon of olive oil and put it in a baking dish. Bake for 25 minutes.

After taking it out of the oven, gently remove the skin from the top. Coat with the tomato sauce and but back in the oven for ten minutes.

✱ The ideal side dish is braised fennel. Cook the bulbs in salted water for 40 minutes. Drain them. Cut them in half and sauté them in a pan with olive oil until they are slightly caramelized.

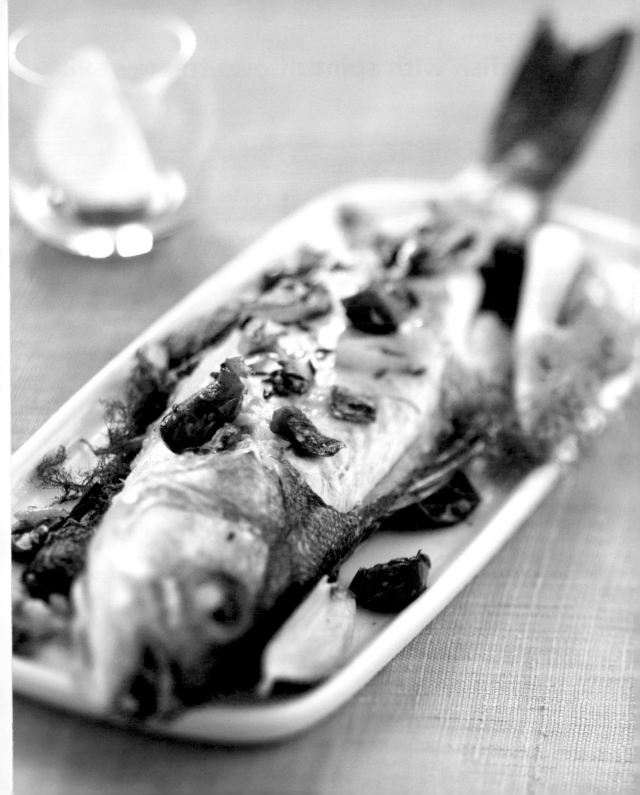

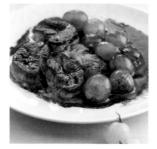

Foie gras sautéed with grapes

Serves 4

■ **Preparation time:**
20 minutes
■ **Cooking time:**
5 minutes

■ **Ingredients:**
> 21oz (600 g) of large green grapes (like Muscat)
> 4 escallops of raw foie gras around 4oz (120 g)
> 1 tablespoon of balsamic vinegar
> 5fl oz (15 cl) pineau des Charentes
> Sel de Guérande
> Freshly ground pepper

Wash the grapes. Peel three quarters of them and eliminate as many seeds as possible. Squeeze the rest to obtain the juice. Set aside. Remove the escallops, season lightly with salt and pepper on both sides. Preheat the oven to 80 °C. Heat a non-stick pan over a high flame and without any grease or oil. The pan must be very hot. Cook the foie gras scallops 30 to 45 seconds on each side in order to caramelize them. Remove them from the pan and put them on a plate on paper towels. Put them in the oven until serving.

Remove 90% of the cooking fat. Deglaze the pan with balsamic vinegar and pineau. Let it reduce for 1 minute over a medium flame, then add the grape juice. Increase the flame to bring the liquid to a boil. Let it reduce by one quarter. Add the peeled grapes and let them heat over a medium flame for around 2 minutes. Season with salt and pepper.

Serve the foie gras escallops in the middle of a warm plate. Pour the sauce around them and arrange the grapes.

✱ Foie gras is not just a festive food with a high gastronomical value. It also has a remarkable nutritional content. It is rich in phosphorous, potassium, magnesium and iron. Its monounsaturated and polyunsaturated essential fatty acids, along with its high folate (B9) content, make it especially favorable for a cardiovascular protection program.

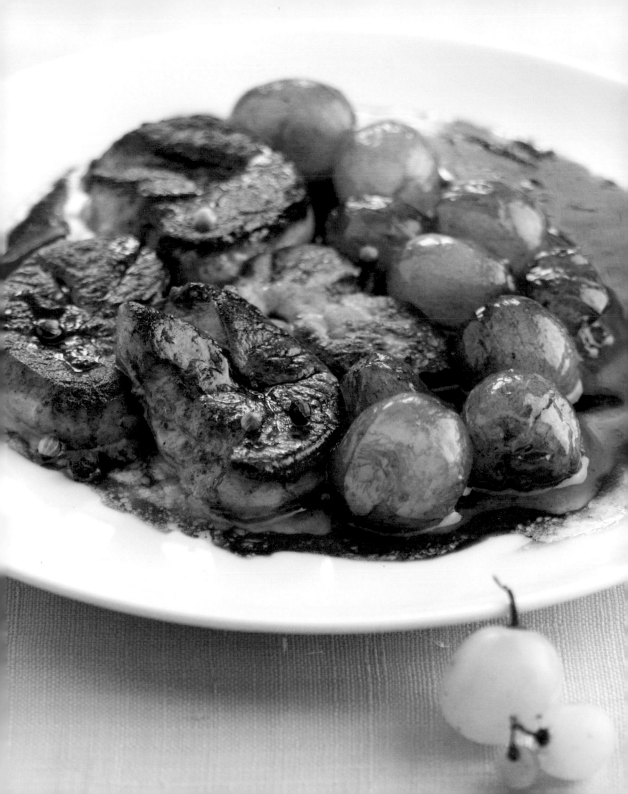

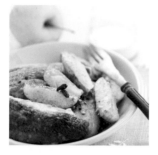

Chicken with apples

Serves 4

■ **Preparation time:**
20 minutes
■ **Cooking time:**
1h30 minutes

■ **Ingredients:**
> 1 free-range chicken
> 4 pinches of
Cayenne pepper
> 2¼ lb (1 kg) of apples
(Granny Smith or golden)
> 1 large tablespoon
of goose (or duck) fat
> 1 teaspoon of powdered
cinnamon
> 18fl oz (50 cl) dry cider
> 1 fat-free chicken
bouillon cube
> 9fl oz (25 cl) low-fat
whipping cream
(or soy cream)
> Salt and pepper

Preheat the oven to 200 °C.

Put the chicken in a baking dish. Season with salt and pepper. Sprinkle with a little Cayenne pepper in the thigh joints. Bake for 1 h 30 minutes.

Peel the apples, cut into quarters and remove the core. Cut the quarters in half widthwise.

In a large frying pan, melt the goose fat, and sauté the apples stirring with a spatula. Sprinkle with cinnamon. Season with salt. The apples are cooked when they are golden brown and soft. Avoid mashing them. Set aside.

Half through cooking the chicken, sprinkle with cider. Keep a large glass for the sauce. In a pan, dissolve the chicken bouillon cube with the glass of cider. Set aside.

When the chicken is cooked, cut it in the baking dish and keep all of the cooking juice. Take all the juice and pour it in the bouillon pan. Reduce if necessary. Add the whipping cream and heat over a low flame. Adjust the seasoning and pour into a sauceboat which has been heated first by running it under very hot water.

Reheat the apples and serve hot.

✱ If using soy cream, heat the sauce before adding, since it does not withstand cooking.

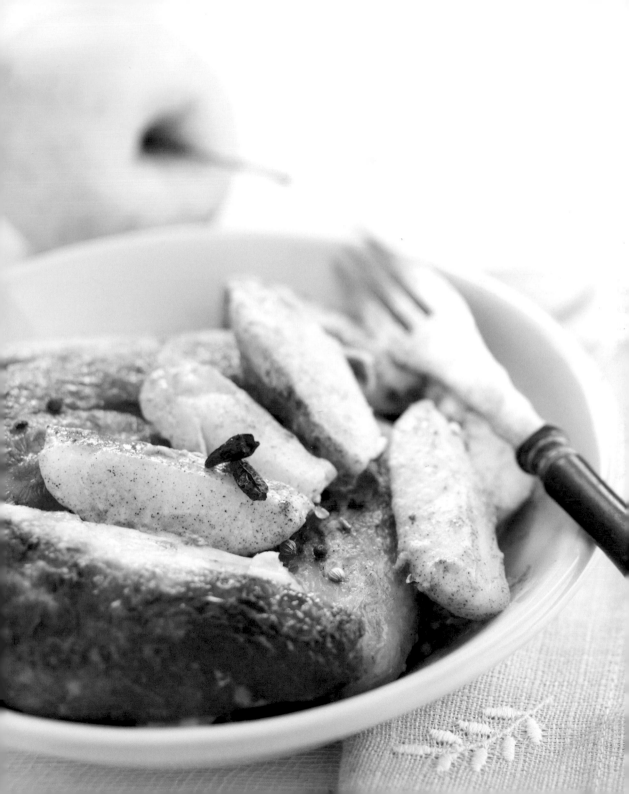

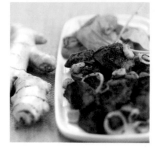

Chicken livers sautéed in ginger

Serves 4

■ **Preparation time:**
5 minutes
■ **Cooking time:**
15 minutes

■ **Ingredients:**
> 3 onions
> A piece of fresh
ginger of almost 1 inch
> A few sprigs of fresh
coriander, chopped
> 2 tablespoons of olive oil
> 1lb (500 g) of chicken
livers
> Salt and pepper

Chop the onions. Peel the ginger and grate it.
Chop the sprigs of fresh coriander.

Brown the onions with the olive oil in a frying pan over
a low flame. When the onions are soft, add the chicken
livers. Cook over a low flame for ten minutes, turning
the pieces over to sear them well on all sides. Season
with salt and pepper.

Add the grated ginger and the coriander, continue
cooking for 4 or 5 minutes and stirring.

Serve hot with a nice green salad.

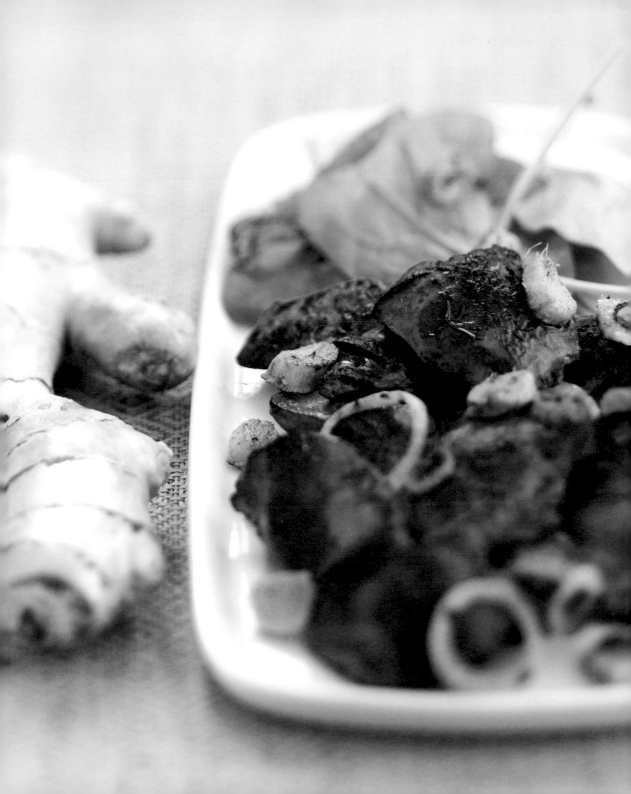

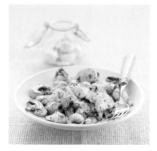

Chicken breast with curry

Serves 4

■ **Preparation time:**
15 minutes
■ **Cooking time:**
15 minutes

■ **Ingredients:**
> 3 onions
> 2 tablespoons of olive oil
> 1 can of sliced
champignons (14oz - 400 g)
> 4 chicken breasts
> 1 knob of goose fat
(or olive oil)
> 1 tablespoon of
curry powder
> 9fl oz (25 cl) low-fat
liquid cream
> Salt and pepper

Slice the onions and brown them in a pot over a low flame in the olive oil until they become very tender. Turn off the burner and set aside.

Drain the champignons in a strainer.

Cut the chicken breasts into 2 to 3 cm chunks. Melt the goose fat in a pan and brown the chicken breast pieces for a few minutes over a very low flame turning them so that they are seared on each side. Season with salt and pepper. Sprinkle half the curry on the meat. Mix and pour in a pot.

Add the onions, champignons, then the liquid cream and the rest of the curry. Mix everything and cook covered for 3 minutes then uncovered for another 3 or 4 minutes for thicken the sauce.

✱ In phase I, this dish should be served with quinoa. In phase II, it can be served with basmati rice or brown rice.

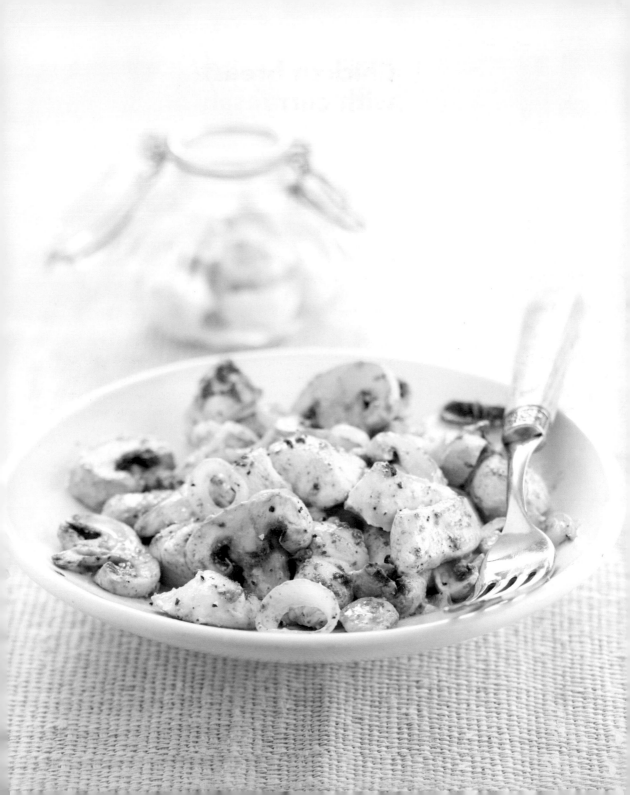

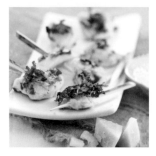

Chicken breast with parmesan

Serves 4

■ **Preparation time:**
15 minutes
■ **Cooking time:**
20 minutes

■ **Ingredients:**
> 5 chicken breasts
(or turkey)
> 1 teaspoon of
powdered thyme
> 3 tablespoons of olive oil
> 2 garlic cloves crushed in
a mortar or press.
> 1 whole yogurt
> 1 bunch chopped parsley
> 7oz (200 g) grated
parmesan
> Salt and pepper

Cut the chicken breasts into 2 by 4 cm chunks. Season with salt and pepper and sprinkle with a little thyme.

Pour 3 tablespoons of olive oil in a large bowl. Add the crushed garlic and yogurt. Whisk. Then add the chopped parsley. Season with salt and pepper. Add the chicken breasts and mix. Preheat the oven to 200 °C.

Put the parmesan in a soup bowl. Roll each piece of chicken in the parmesan. Put them on the bottom of an oiled baking pan. The pieces can be next to each other but not overlapping.

If there is still some parmesan, spread it uniformly over the surface of the chicken pieces.
Bake 15 to 20 minutes, until the chicken is cooked.

Serve with a large green salad dressed with vinaigrette provençale (see the vinaigrette recipe on pg. 78)

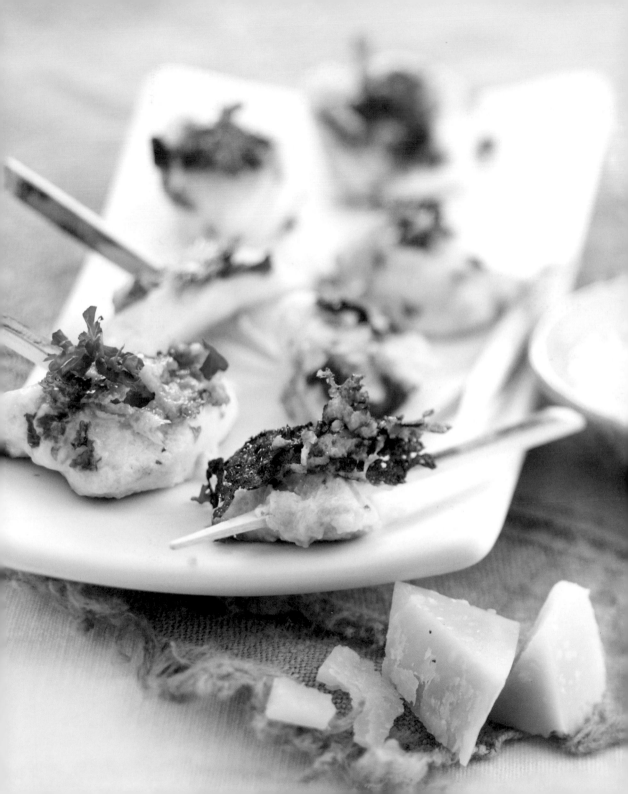

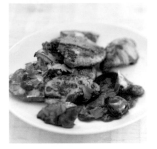

Foies de volaille à la provençale

Serves 4

■ **Preparation time:**
5 minutes
■ **Cooking time:**
15 minutes

■ **Ingredients:**
> 4 garlic cloves
> 4oz (125 g) tomato paste
> Glass dry white wine
> 1 tablespoon
of goose fat
> 21oz (600 g) of dressed
chicken livers
> 1/2 teaspoon of
herbes de Provence
> 3 sprigs Italian parsley
> Salt and pepper

Peel and finely chop the garlic.

Pour the tomato paste in a bowl. Thin it with hot white wine. Season with salt and pepper.

Melt the goose fat in a frying pan. Add the chopped garlic. Brown the chicken livers in the pan turning them so that they are cooked uniformly. Sprinkle the herbes de Provence when you start cooking. Season with salt and pepper and keep warm.

Place the chicken livers on warm individual plates. Coat with tomato sauce. Sprinkle with parsley.

✱ This dish can be served with flageolet beans, green lentils or quinoa.

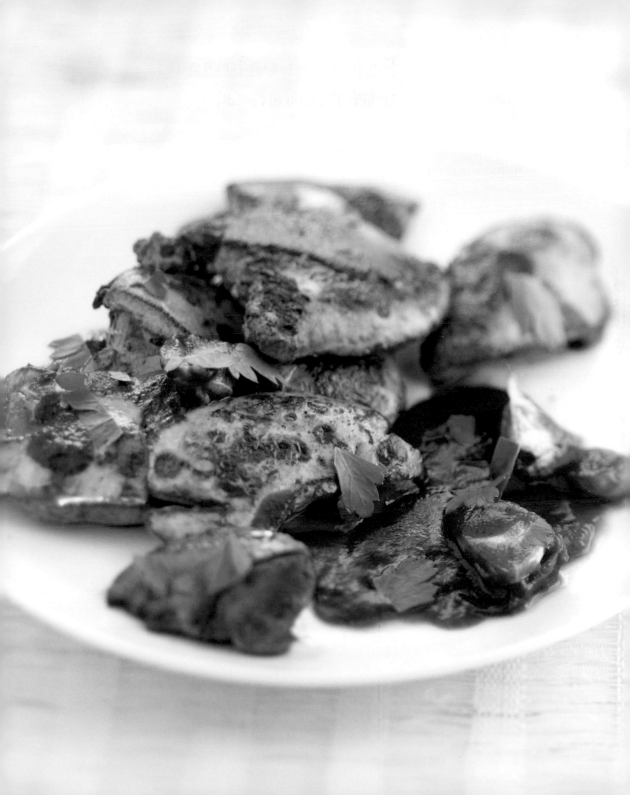

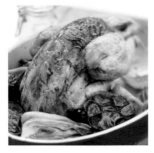

Chicken with pastis and fennel

Serves 4

■ **Preparation time:**
10 minutes
■ **Cooking time:**
1h15 minutes

■ **Ingredients:**
> 1 free-range chicken
3¼ lb (1.5 kg), ready to cook
> 15 garlic cloves
cleaned and peeled
> Olive oil
> ½ glass of pastis
> 1 pinch of Cayenne pepper
> 1 teaspoon of
herbes de Provence
> 7oz (200 g) pitted
black olives
> 4 fennel bulbs
> 1 knob of goose fat
> Salt and freshly
ground pepper

Preheat the oven to 200 °C. Season with the interior of the chicken with salt and pepper. Add 5 garlic cloves.

Put the chicken on a large platter. Generously coat all the sides with olive oil. Sprinkle with pastis. Season with salt and pepper. Add the Cayenne pepper and sprinkle with herbes de Provence. Place the remaining garlic cloves on the platter around then chicken and then the black olives. Bake 1 h 15. In the meantime, baste the chicken three of four times with its cooking juice, adding hot water if necessary.

During this time, cook the fennel bulbs in salted water for 40 minutes. Drain them, cut them in half lengthwise and sauté them in a pan with goose fat until they are golden brown. Place them on the platter around the chicken for the last 15 minutes of cooking.

Cut the chicken on its platter in order to keep as much of the juice as possible. Arrange the pieces on a warm serving plate or, even better, serve in the cooking platter.

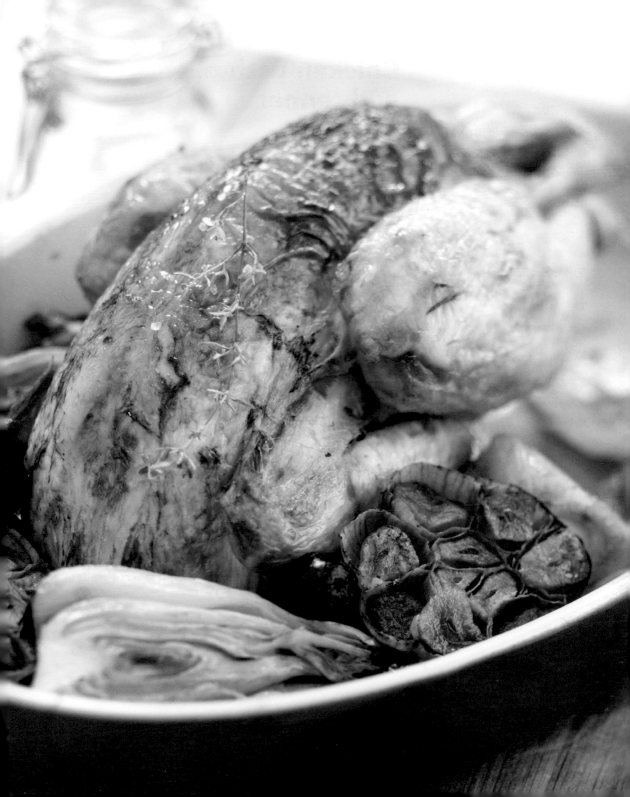

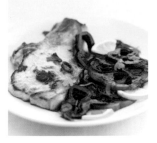

Veal chops with two bell peppers

Serves 4

■ **Preparation time:**
15 minutes
■ **Cooking time:**
1h10 minutes

■ **Ingredients:**
> 2 green bell peppers
and 2 red bell peppers
> 5 tablespoons of olive oil
> 6 ripe tomatoes
> 3 garlic cloves
> 3 shallots
> 1 glass of very tanniny
red wine (côtes-du-rhône
or corbières)
> 1 teaspoon of mild
paprika powder
> 4 veal chops 7oz
(200 g) each
> 1 knob of goose fat
> 3 sprigs Italian parsley
> 2 lemons
> Salt and pepper

Cut the bell peppers in half. Remove everything that is inside: peduncle, seeds and white filaments. Drop them in boiling water for 10 minutes. Drain them and cut them into 2 by 4 cm chunks. Sauté them with 2 to 3 tablespoons of olive oil in a frying pan. Let them cook over a medium flame for 20 to 25 minutes, stirring regularly.

Drop the tomatoes into boiling water and cook for 40 seconds then rinse under cold water. Peel them and slice them in quarters. Remove the seeds and keep the pulp. Set aside. Peel the garlic and shallots. Chop them finely.

Sauté the garlic and shallots in another pan containing 2 tablespoons of olive oil. Add the tomato pulp and red wine. Season with salt and pepper and let simmer for 15 minutes. Add the peppers to the tomato sauce. Season with the paprika. Set aside.

Season the two sides of the veal chop with salt and pepper. Melt the goose fat in a frying pan. When it is very hot, brown the veal chops 8 minute on each side. During this time, chop half of the parsley.

Arrange the chops on a platter or individual plates. Pour the sauce around them. Garnish with lemons cut in half and sprinkle with chopped and whole parsley.

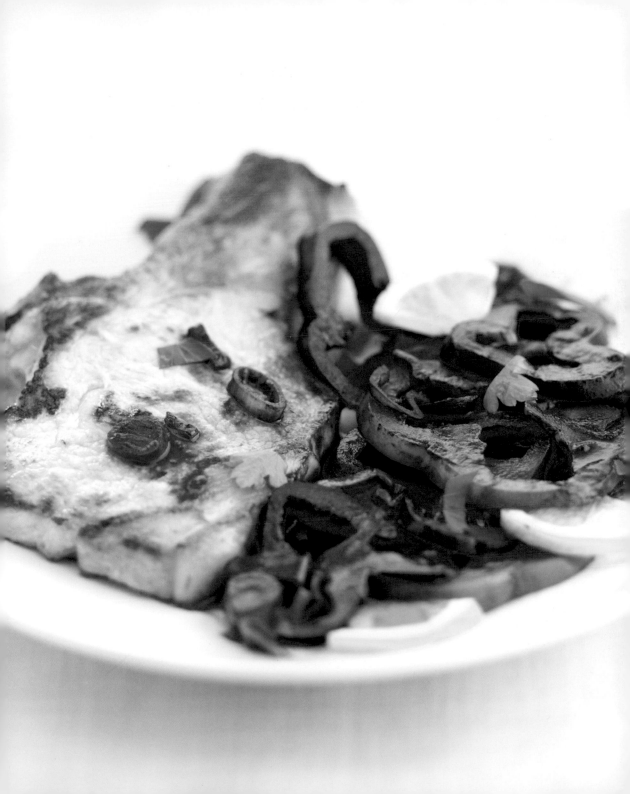

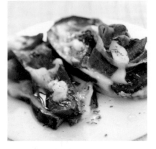

Croque-aubergine

Serves 4

■ **Preparation time:**
15 minutes
■ **Cooking time:**
20 minutes
■ **Standing time:**
30 minutes

■ **Ingredients:**
> 2 large eggplants
> Olive oil
> 8 slices of prosciutto
> 8 to 10 slices of
processed cheese slices
> Herbes de Provence
> Fresh basil
> Salt and pepper

Preheat the oven to 200 °C.

Cut the eggplants lengthwise into 1 cm thick slices. Remove the excess moisture by covering all sides with salt and letting them stand 30 minutes. Brown them on both sides with plenty of olive oil in a frying pan. Slightly season with salt and pepper and set aside.

Put the prosciutto slices into the pan for a few seconds.

Put the eggplant slices on the bottom of a baking pan. Arrange the prosciutto on top. Complete the sandwich by placing the processed cheese slices. Sprinkle with herbes de Provence. Bake for 10 to 15 minutes, enough time to let the cheese melt.

Serve garnishing with basil leaves.

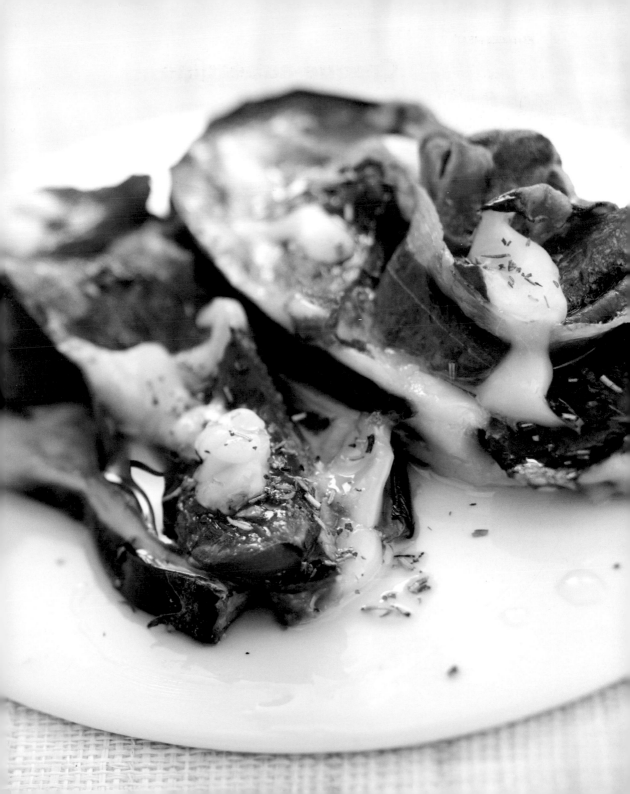

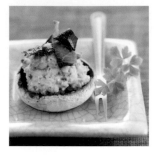

Stuffed champignons

Serves 4

■ **Preparation time:**
20 minutes
■ **Cooking time:**
35 minutes

■ **Ingredients:**
> 12 very large champignons
> 2 onions finely chopped
> 2 tablespoons of olive oil
> 2 crushed garlic cloves
> 2oz (50 g) prosciutto
(without fat) chopped finely
> 3½ oz (100 g) chicken
breast chopped finely
> 2fl oz (5 cl) of fat-free
chicken stock
> 2 tablespoons
of grated parmesan
> 2 tablespoons of
chopped parsley
> Salt and pepper

Remove the end of the champignons. Gently peel the cap starting from the ring. Chop the stalk after having removed the dirty end.

In a frying pan, brown the onions in the olive oil until they become very soft. Add the chopped champignon stalks and garlic. Stir for at least a minute. Add the prosciutto, chicken and enough bouillon to moisten everything. Season with salt and pepper.

Preheat the oven to 190 °C. Stuff the mushrooms and place them on a baking dish. Drizzle with plenty of olive oil on each mushroom. Sprinkle with parmesan. Bake 20 to 30 minutes.

Serve hot on a bed of lettuce after sprinkling with parsley.

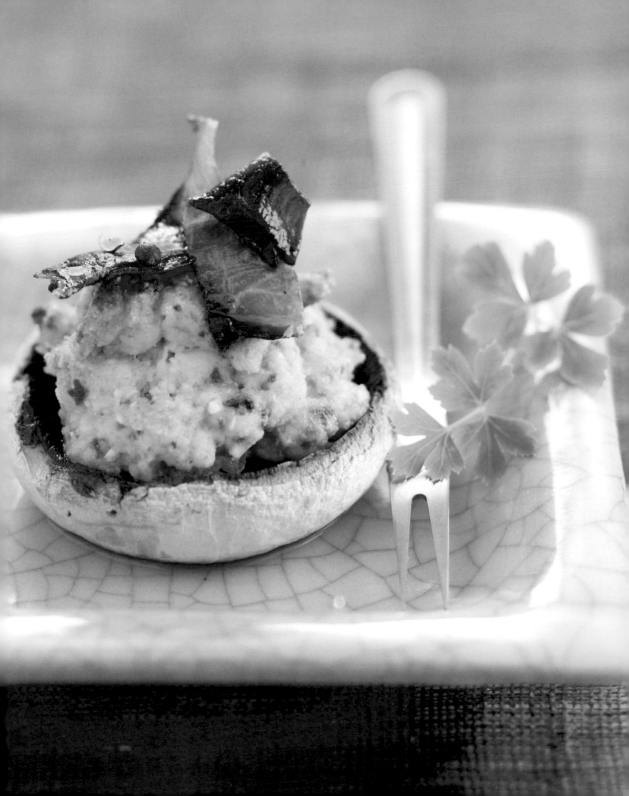

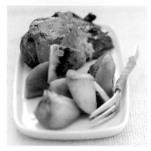

Confit of duck with apples

Serves 4

■ **Preparation time:**
20 minutes
■ **Cooking time:**
45 minutes

■ **Ingredients:**
> 1 can of confit of duck containing 4 thighs
> 12 Granny Smith apples
> Powdered cinnamon
> A few sprigs Italian parsley
> Salt and pepper

Preheat the oven to 80 °C. Open the can of confit. Take out 5 tablespoons of fat. Put the can in the oven and wait until the fat completely melts.

During this time, peel the apples. Cut them in quarters and remove the core, then cut each quarter in half.

Let the 5 tablespoon of duck fat melt in a large non-stick pan. Sauté the pieces of apple over a medium flame stirring often. Season with salt and pepper and generously sprinkle with cinnamon. Continue cooking until the apples become soft. They should be slightly caramelized, but not burnt. Thus the flame needs to be adjusted.

When the fat in the can is completely melted, take the thighs out carefully and arrange them on a plate to let the grease run off. Arrange them (skin side up) on a baking dish. Turn on the broiler and let them cook for 10 to 15 minutes 20 cm under the broiler. The skin on the thighs may be slightly grilled, but the meat should not dry out.

Put the thighs on individual plates, put the apples around them and garnish with Italian parsley.

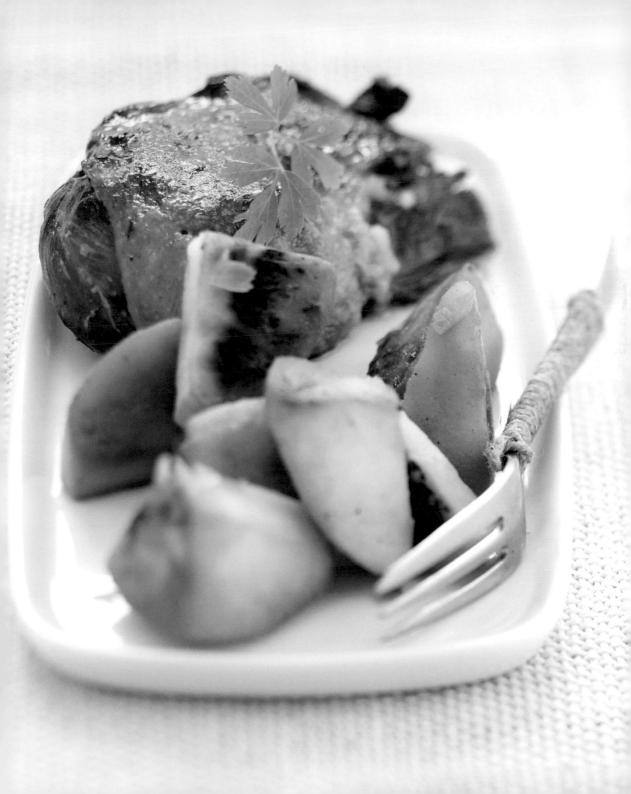

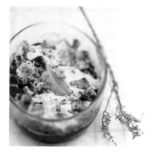

Eggplant gratin with bacon cubes

Serves 4

■ **Preparation time:**
30 minutes
■ **Cooking time:**
1 hour
■ **Standing time:**
20 minutes

■ **Ingredients:**
> 5 small eggplants
> Olive oil
> 4 large onions
> 3½ oz (100 g) of very thin (julienne) bacon cubes
> 1 small jar of tomato paste (4½ lb - 140 g)
> 5oz (150 g) grated gruyere
> 2 mozzarella balls
> Herbes de Provence
> Salt and pepper

Cut the eggplants in thin slices 0.5 cm thick. Salt both sides and remove the excess moisture for 20 minutes. Dry them with paper towels, then slightly coat them with olive oil using a brush. Sauté them in a large pan (or on a "flattop grill") and let them cook over a low flame until they become golden brown and very soft. Be careful not to let them burn.

Peel the onions and chop them. Brown them over a low flame in olive oil until they become transparent and very soft. Put them on paper towels.

Sauté the bacon over a low flame to make them release as much of their fat as possible without burning them. Set aside after cooking and put them on paper towels.

Dry the eggplant with paper towels. Cover the bottom of a large baking dish with the eggplant slices, like for the bottom of a pie. The slices can be overlapping on two or three levels.

Spread the tomato paste uniformly over the fried eggplants. Divide the onions over the entire surface. Do the same thing with the bacon, then cover with grated gruyere.

Cut the mozzarella balls into thin slices, in order to cover the entire surface of the dish. Lightly season with salt. Season with pepper and sprinkle with herbes de Provence. Place under the broiler until the mozzarella is completely melted.

Serve hot with a nice green salad.

✱ This gratin can also be made in individual plates.

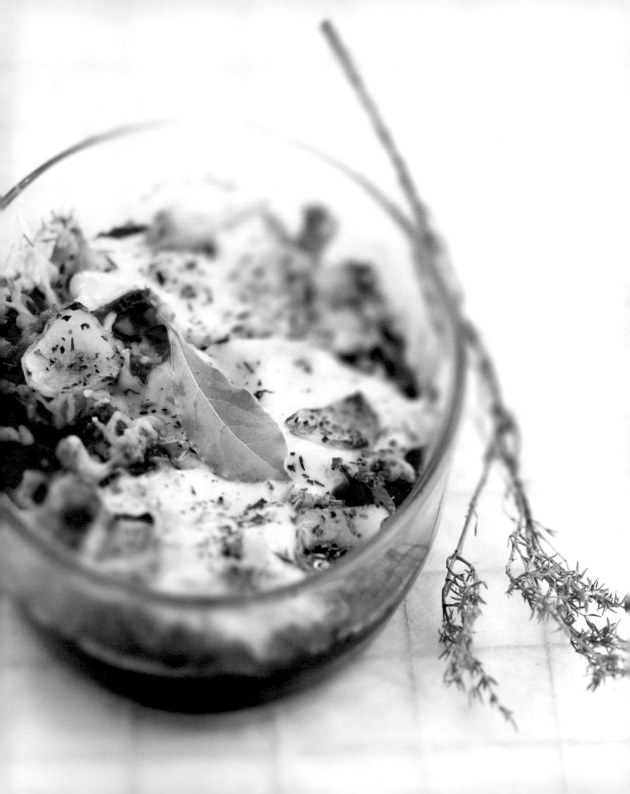

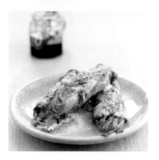

Endive gratin with ham

Serves 4

■ **Preparation time:**
5 minutes
■ **Cooking time:**
45 minutes

■ **Ingredients:**
> 4 endives
> 8 slices of white ham
> Olive oil
> 10fl oz (30 cl) low-fat liquid crème fraîche
> 7oz (200 g) grated gruyere
> A few basil parsley (for the garnish)
> Salt and pepper

Cut the end of the endives. Eliminate the damaged leaves. Place them in the basket of a steamer and cook for 30 minutes. Drain and let them cool. Cut them in half and let them drain again. Season with salt and pepper.

Roll the half endives in a slice of ham. Put them on the bottom of a baking pan previously oiled with olive oil. Preheat the oven to 200 °C.

Pour the liquid cream and two thirds of the grated gruyere in a bowl. Mix energetically until obtaining a type of very uniform béchamel. Pour this over the endives. Add the rest of the gruyere to the top. Bake for 10 to 15 minutes, enough time so that the top becomes golden brown.

Garnish with sprigs of parsley.

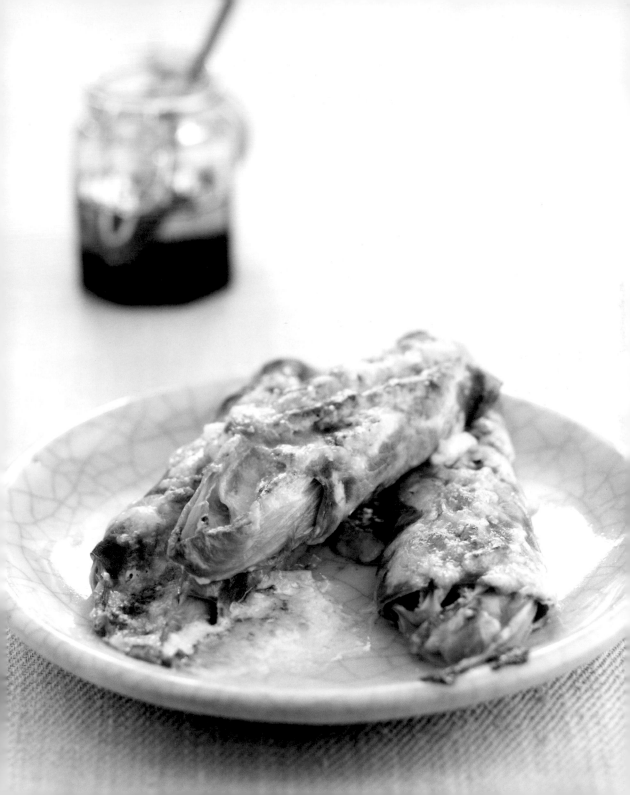

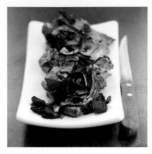

Entrecôte marchand de vin

Serves 4

■ **Preparation time:**
5 minutes
■ **Cooking time:**
20 minutes

■ **Ingredients:**
> 10 shallots
> 2 knob of goose fat
> 9fl oz (25 cl) of very
tanniny red wine (corbières)
> 2 thick rib steaks
14oz (400 g) each
> 1 bunch chopped parsley
> Salt and pepper

Peel the shallots and chop finely. Sauté them in a pan over a low flame with a large knob of goose fat. Add the wine. Let it reduce until the sauce becomes creamy. Season with salt and pepper and keep warm over a very low flame.

In another pan melt a knob of goose fat. Cook the steaks over a high flame for 2 to 4 minutes on each side, based on the thickness and how well done you want it. Rib steaks are normally eaten rare.

Cut the steak into 3 cm slices along the width. Divide them on hot individual plates. Coat with the sauce and garnish with parsley.

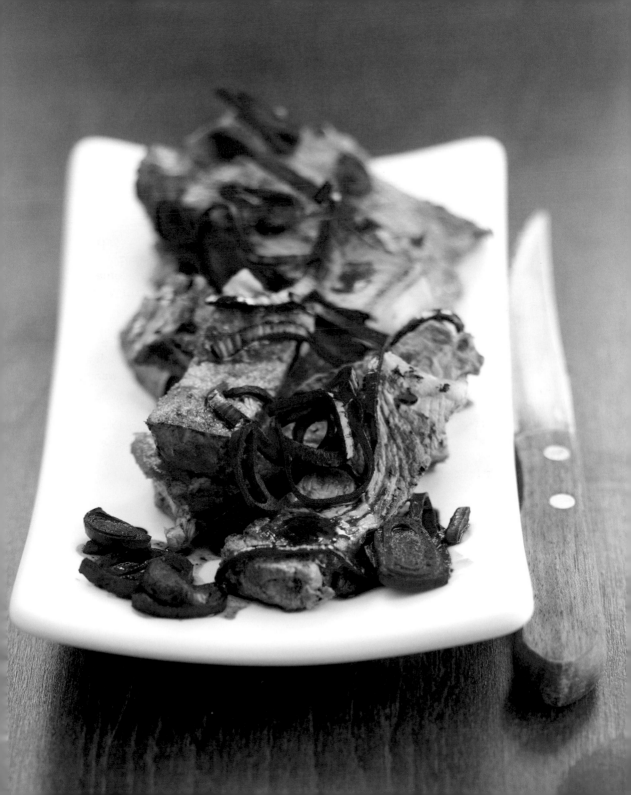

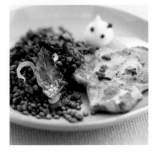

Pork chops
with green lentils

Serves 4

■ **Preparation time:**
5 minutes
■ **Cooking time:**
40 minutes

■ **Ingredients:**
> 1 liter of fat-free
chicken stock
> 1 large onion
> 1 knob of goose fat
> 6 pork chops
> 5oz (150 g) small bacon
cubes, unsmoked
> 1lb (500 g) Du Puy
green lentils
> 1 small onion studded
with cloves
> 1 bouquet garni
> Salt and pepper

Prepare the stock in a pot. Chop the onion.

Melt 1 knob of goose fat in a non-stick frying pan.
Brown the pork chops over a high flame for 1 minute on
each side. Set aside. In the same pan and with the same
fat, sauté the onion and bacon.

Put the lentils into the stock. Add the onions and the
bacon without their cooking fat. Then add the studded
onion and the bouquet garni. Arrange the pork chops
on the top. Simmer covered for 30 to 35 minutes.
The lentils should be tender but not pureed. Add the
seasoning at the end of cooking.

Before serving remove the studded onion and the
bouquet garni.

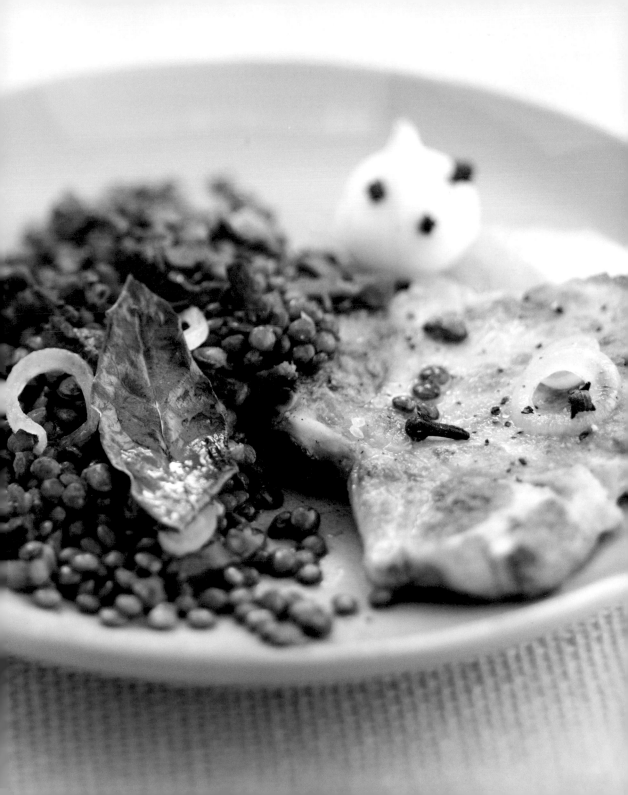

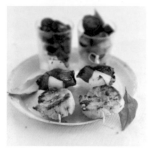

Filet mignon
skewers with prunes

Serves 4

■ **Preparation time:**
20 minutes
■ **Cooking time:**
10 minutes

■ **Ingredients:**
> 12 pitted prunes
> 7fl oz (20 cl) white wine
> 1 pork filet mignon
> 4 medium size onions
> 12 slices smoked bacon
> 8 bay leaves
> 1 dash of olive oil.
> Herbes de Provence
> Salt and pepper

Poach the prunes over a low flame for 5 minutes in the white wine. Turn off the flame. Cover and let swell for 10 minutes.

Cut the filet mignon into a dozen cubes.

Peel the onions and cut them in quarters.

Drain the prunes. Wrap each prune in a slice of bacon.

Make skewers by alternating: the bay leaves, the meat cubes, the onion quarters, the prunes with bacon. Sprinkle a little olive oil. Season with salt and pepper and sprinkle with herbes de Provence.

Cook on a grill 5 minutes on each side.

✱ This dish can be served with Montignac ratatouille (see the recipe pg. 212).

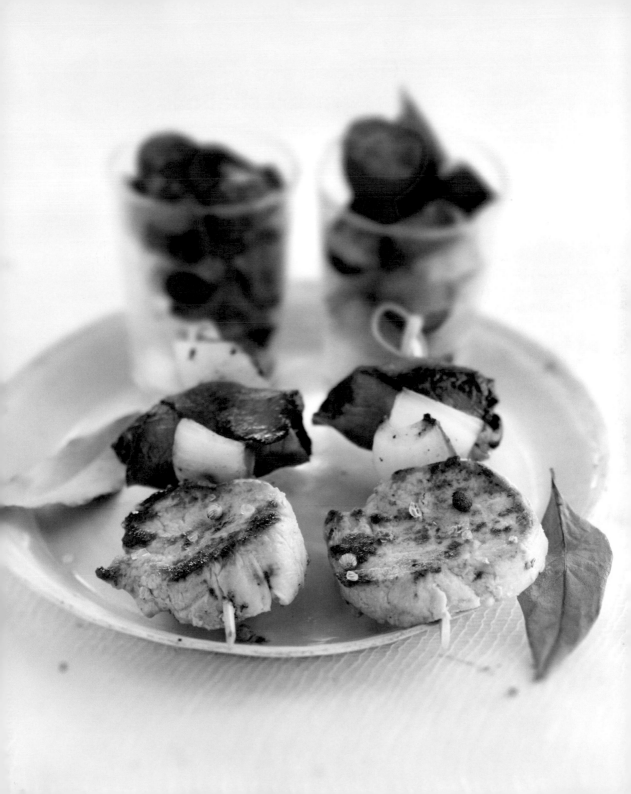

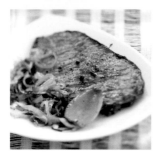

Hanger steak on grated shallots

Serves 4

■ **Preparation time:**
12 minutes
■ **Cooking time:**
15 minutes

■ **Ingredients:**
> 21oz (600 g) of shallots
> 2 tablespoons of goose fat
> 4 hanger steaks 7oz
(200 g) each
> Italian parsley
> Salt and pepper

Preheat the oven to 100 °C.

Peel the shallots. Cut them into thin slices. In a large frying pan melt the goose fat and sauté the shallots over a very low flame stirring with a spatula until they turn brown, but without letting them burn. Season with salt and pepper. Remove them from the pan with skimmer and put them on paper towels to remove the grease. Keep in a hot oven and divide onto 4 individual plates.

In the same pan and in the same cooking grease, brown the hanger steaks over a high flame for 1 to 2 minutes on each side based on the thickness and how done you want them. Hanger steak is eaten rare, even very rare for those who like it. Season with salt and pepper.

Remove the plates from the oven and put the steaks on the grated shallots. Garnish with parsley.

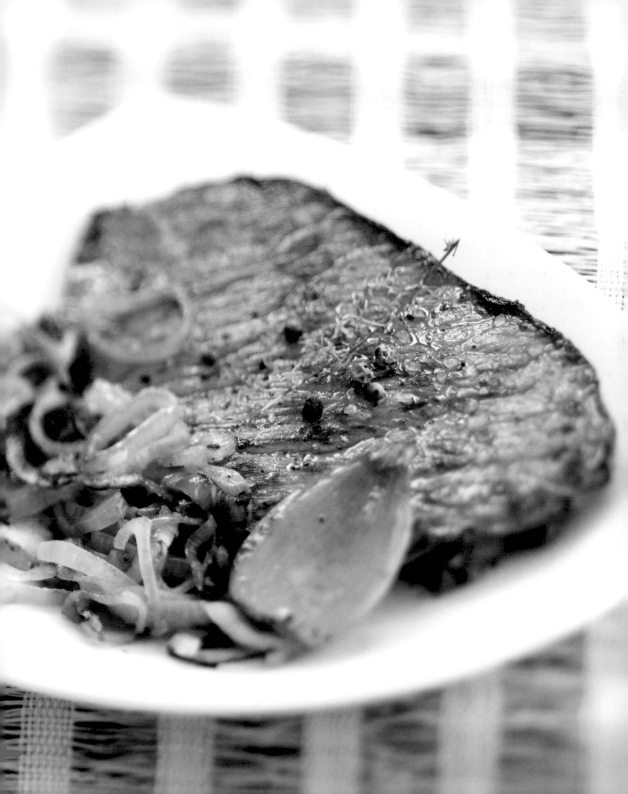

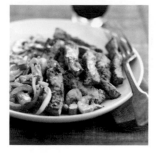

Beef with paprika

Serves 4

■ **Preparation time:**
15 minutes
■ **Cooking time:**
15 minutes

■ **Ingredients:**
> 2 large onions
> 1 knob of goose fat
> 1/2 can of sliced
champignons (3¾ oz - 110 g)
> 1lb (500 g) of lean beef,
in the round
> 3½ oz (100 g) of chopped
cornichons
> 1 tablespoon of paprika
> 2 pinches of
Cayenne pepper
> 5fl oz (15 cl) red wine
> 5fl oz (15 cl) low-fat
crème fraîche
> Salt and pepper

Peel the onions and chop them. Sauté them in a large pan with the goose fat. Add the champignons. Let them cook 2 minutes and then pour into a pot leaving the cooking grease in the pan.

Cut the beef into slices 5 to 6 cm long by 1 cm. Brown them in the onion pan for 1 minute stirring well and adding a little goose fat if necessary. Season with salt and pepper. Pour in the pot.

Place the pot on a low flame, add the chopped cornichons, paprika and Cayenne pepper. Moisten with the red wine. Let cook for 3 minute while stirring.
Add the crème fraîche and let cook another 3 minutes. Serve hot.

★ This dish can be served with broccoli, cauliflower or Brussels sprouts.

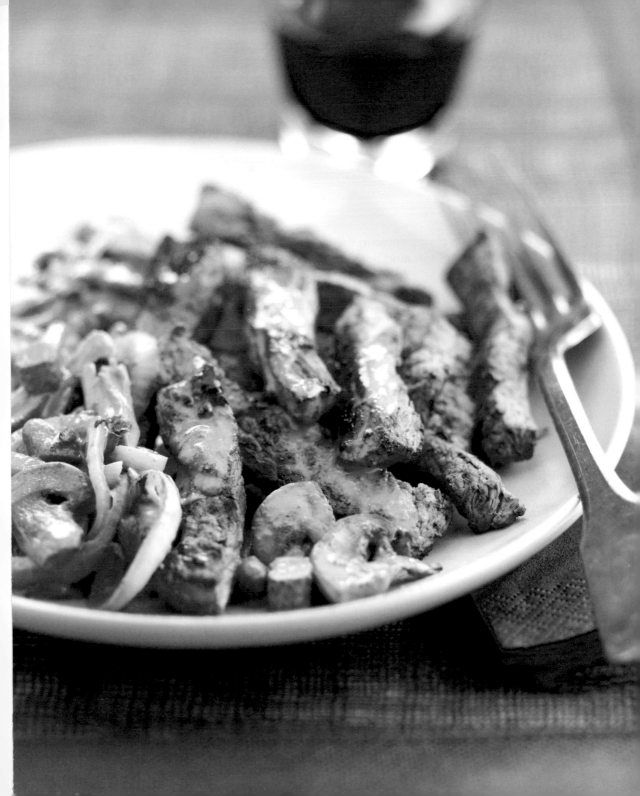

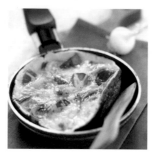

Omelet with eggplants

Serves 4

■ **Preparation time:**
20 minutes

■ **Standing time:**
1 hour

■ **Cooking time:**
45 minutes

■ **Ingredients:**
> 1 large eggplant
> 3 medium size tomatoes
> 1/2 tablespoon of olive oil
> 1 chopped onion
> 6 large eggs
> 7oz (200 g) grated gruyere
> Salt and pepper

Cut the eggplant in large pieces, approximately 2 cm by 2 cm. Steam them for 30 to 35 minutes. The pieces are cooked when they are very soft, even mushy, and they have turned brown. After they have cooked, put them in a large strainer and let them drain for at least an hour.

Boil the tomatoes for 40 seconds then rinse under cold water. Peel them and then empty them, keep the pulp cut into small pieces. Drain on paper towels.

Turn on the broiler and put the rack in the upper part.

Heat a little olive oil in a large pan. Sauté the chopped onions until they become very soft. During this time, beat the eggs in a bowl. Season with salt and pepper. Pour the beaten eggs in the pan on the onions. Add the eggplants and tomatoes and uniformly divide them over the entire surface of the pan. Gently stir to obtain a uniform cooking. Slightly season with salt and pepper.

Off the flame, spread the gruyere uniformly over the entire omelet. Place the pan under the broiler and leave the door open to keep the handle outside and check the cooking. As soon as the cheese becomes browned remove the pan from the oven and serve hot with a seasonal salad.

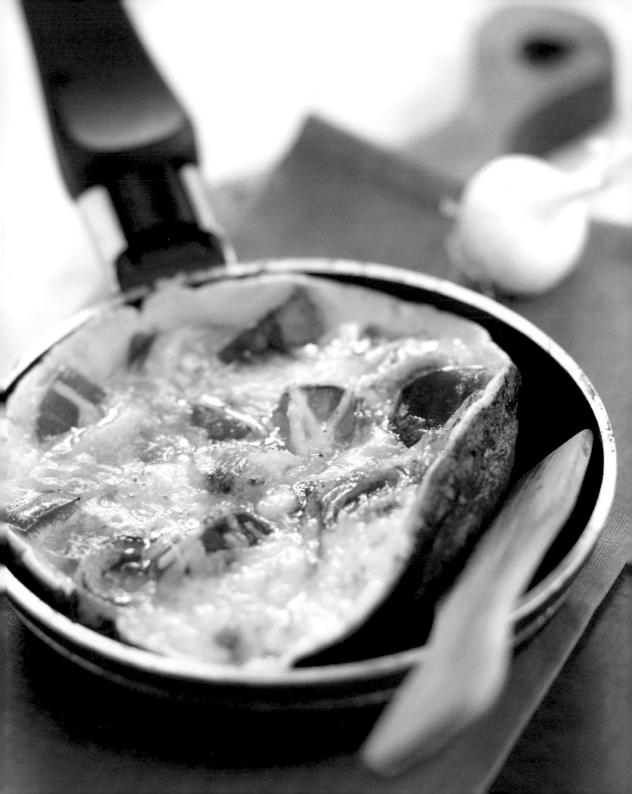

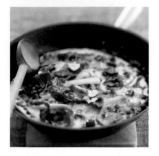

Vegetable omelet with chorizo

Serves 4

■ **Preparation time:**
15 minutes
■ **Cooking time:**
10 minutes

■ **Ingredients:**
> 1 onion
> 2 garlic cloves
> 1 red bell pepper
> 2oz (50 g) peas (canned)
> 4 jarred asparagus
> 2oz (50 g) of champignon mushrooms (canned)
> 7oz (200 g) prosciutto
> 3½ oz (100 g) chorizo
> 1 artichoke heart
> 2 tablespoons of olive oil
> 8 large fresh eggs
> 2 sprigs Italian parsley
> Salt and pepper

Peel and chop the onion. Chop the garlic.

Cut the bell pepper in half. Deseed it and cut into small pieces.

Open the cans of peas and champignons and the jar of asparagus. Drain them in a strainer.

Cut the prosciutto into thin slices and the chorizo into rounds. Cut the asparagus into 2 cm lengths. Cut the artichoke heart into small pieces.

In a frying pan, sauté the chopped onion and the bell pepper pieces in 1 tablespoon of hot olive oil. Constantly mix with a wooden spatula. Add the garlic and the champignons at the end of cooking.

In a bowl, crack the eggs and beat. Season with salt and pepper. Pour the contents into the pan and then add the other ingredients. Mix.

Heat 1 tablespoon of olive oil in a large pan. Pour in the contents of the bowl and cook over a high flame stirring gently with a fork to obtain uniform cooking.

Garnish with Italian parsley and serve hot.

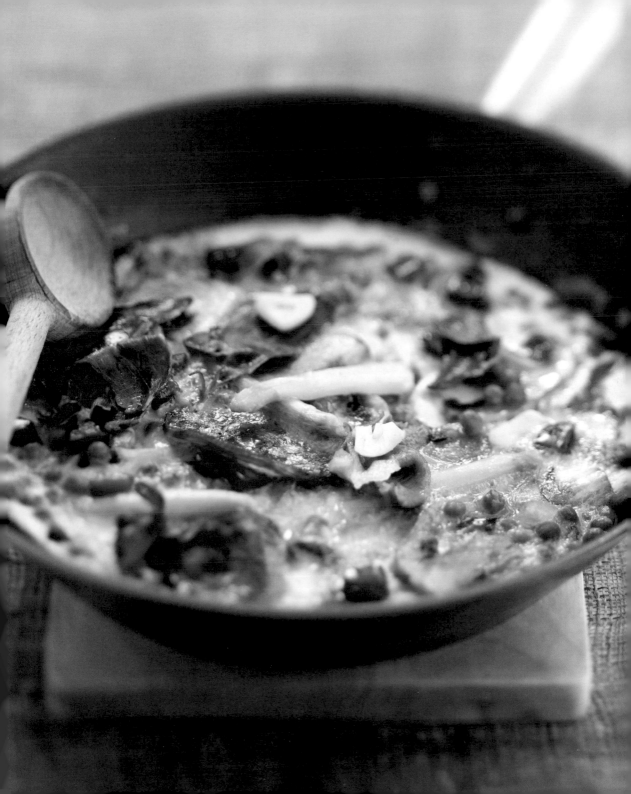

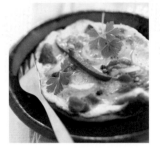

Omelet andalouse

Serves 4

■ **Preparation time:**
10 minutes
■ **Cooking time:**
10 minutes

■ **Ingredients:**
> 5 tomatoes
> 3 large onions
> 2 red bell peppers
> 2 and 1/2 soup
spoons of olive oil
> 8 eggs
> Parsley
> Salt and pepper

Drop the tomatoes into boiling water and cook for 40 seconds then rinse under cold water. Peel them, deseed and cut the flesh into chunks. Keep them in a strainer to let them drain.

Chop the onions. Empty out the peppers then cut them into very thin slices.

Slightly brown the onions with 2 tablespoons of olive oil in a frying pan. Add the peppers and continue cooking over a low flame, stirring regularly. Add the tomatoes. As soon as they are soft, set aside.

Beat the eggs in a salad bowl. Season with salt and pepper. Start heating a frying pan with 1/2 tablespoon of olive oil. When it is hot pour in the eggs and let them set over a high flame for 2 to 3 minutes, mixing everything with a spatula (or fork) so that the omelet cooks uniformly.

When it is a little dry on the edges and still runny in the middle, place half of the vegetable mixture in the middle. Let it cook a second then fold the omelet and slide it onto a long platter.

Arrange the rest of the vegetables at each end and sprinkle with parsley.

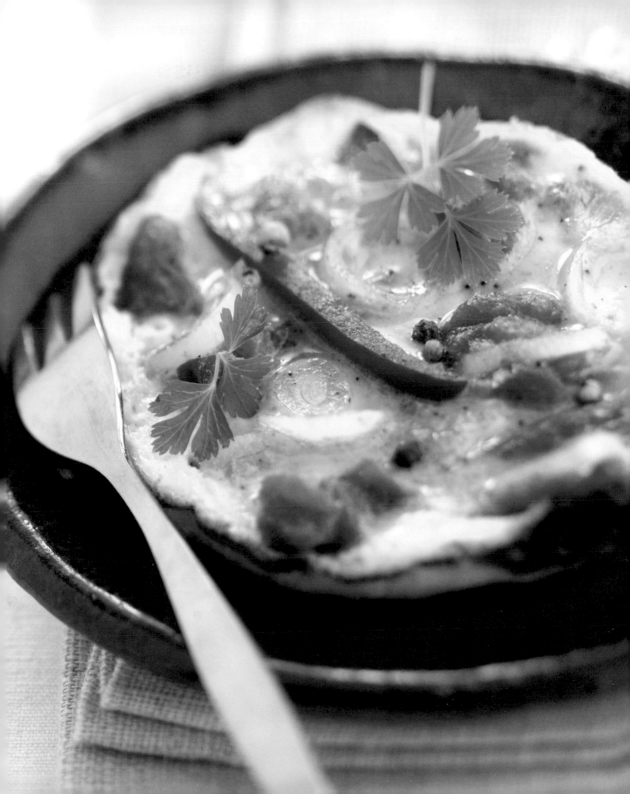

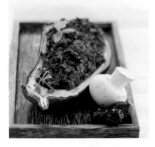

Stuffed eggplants
à la provençale

Serves 4

■ **Preparation time:**
15 minutes
■ **Cooking time:**
50 minutes

■ **Ingredients:**
> 2 medium size eggplants
> Olive oil
> 7oz (200 g) of champignon mushrooms (canned or fresh)
> 2 minced garlic cloves
> 1 tablespoon
of chopped mint
> 1 tablespoon of parsley
> 60 pitted black olives
sliced thinly
> 1 egg
> Salt and freshly ground pepper

Preheat the oven to 210 °C.

Wash the eggplant, cut off the ends and split them in half along the length. With the tip of a knife, carefully crisscross the flesh and avoid piercing the skin. Season with salt and sprinkle with olive oil. Put the eggplants on a baking dish and bake for 30 minutes.

Chop the champignons. In a pan, heat 2 to 3 table-spoons of olive oil, sauté the chopped champignons stirring with a spatula to make them release their moisture. Set aside.

Remove the eggplants from the oven. Using a spoon, remove the pulp from the 4 eggplant halves being careful not to damage the skin. Mash it with a fork to make a coarse puree.

Put the pan back on the flame and add the eggplant pulp. Mix well with a spatula for 1 to 2 minutes and then turn off the burner.

To prepare the stuffing, add the garlic, mint, parsley, black olives and egg, previously beaten with a whisk. Season with salt and pepper. Stir with a spatula to make the mixture uniform.

Stuff the eggplant skins with the stuffing. Put them on an oiled baking dish. Bake for 15 minutes at 210 °C. Serve very hot with a green salad.

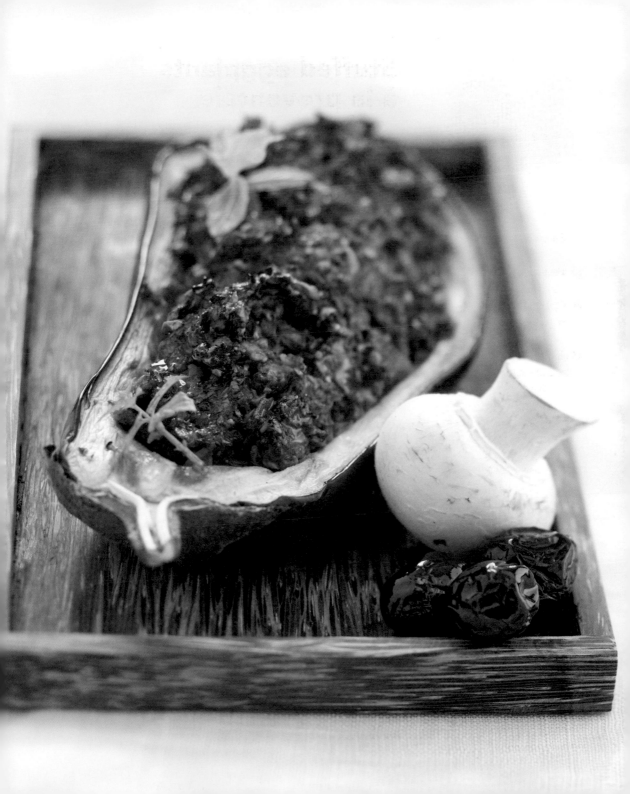

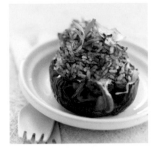

Bell peppers stuffed with basmati rice

Serves 4

■ **Preparation time:**
15 minutes
■ **Cooking time:**
45 minutes

■ **Ingredients:**
> 2 onions
> 4 red bell peppers
> 2oz (50 g) tomato paste
> 14oz (400 g) of cooked basmati rice
> 3 egg whites
> 1 tablespoon of tarragon (fresh or dried)
> 1 tablespoon of cardamom powder
> Salt and pepper

Peel the onions and chop them.
Steam them for 15 minutes.

Wash the bell peppers and completely empty them. Steam them whole for 20 to 25 minutes.

Preheat the oven to 180°C.

Slightly dilute the tomato paste with a little warm water.

In a bowl, mix the cooked rise, tomato paste, onions and scrambled egg whites. Add the tarragon and cardamom. Season with salt and pepper. Mix until obtaining a uniform stuffing.

Fill the bell peppers with this mixture and put them in a baking dish. Bake for 20 minutes.

✱ This dish can be served with a basil tomato sauce (see the recipe pg. 220).

✱ This fat free carbohydrate dish is particularly suited for phase 1.

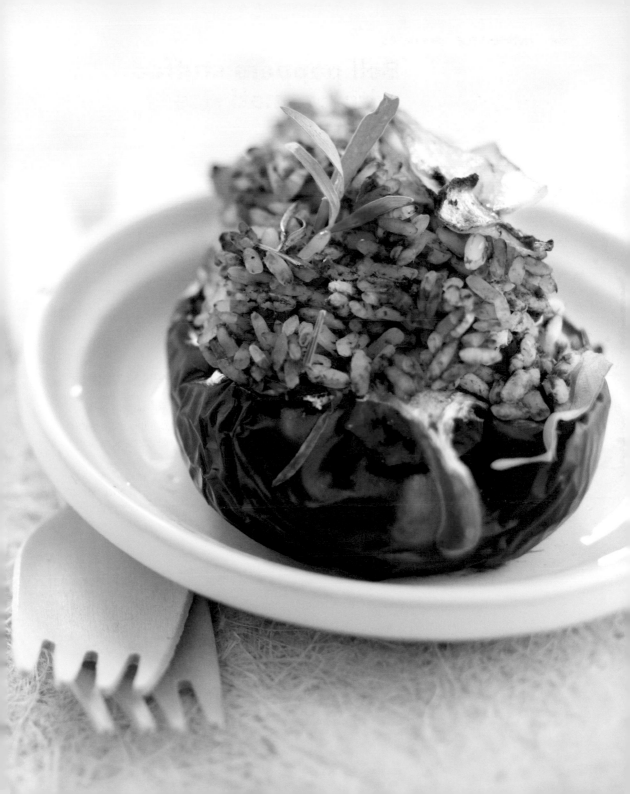

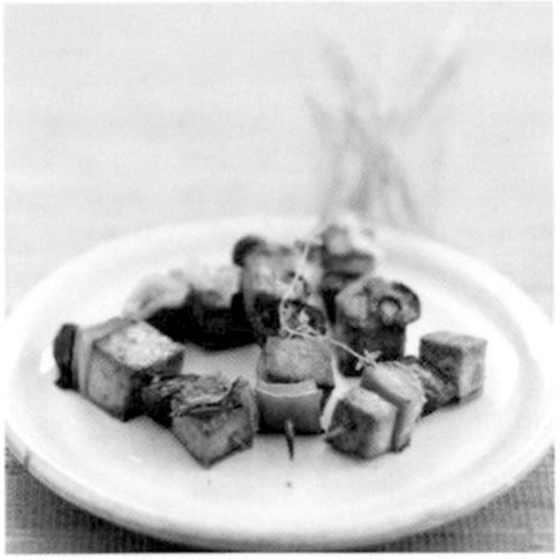

Tofu skewers

Serves 4

■ **Preparation time:**
10 minutes
■ **Cooking time:**
15 minutes

■ **Ingredients:**
> 4 large tomatoes
> 4 medium size onions
> 2 bell peppers
(1 green and 1 red)
> 7oz (200 g) smoked tofu
> 1/2 teaspoon of cumin
> 1/2 teaspoon of nutmeg
> 1 dash of olive oil
(optional)
> Salt

Wash the tomatoes and split them into six.

Peel the onions and cut them into six.

Wash and deseed the bell peppers and cut them into 3 cm by 3 cm squares.

Cut the tofu into cubes.

Insert the pieces on 4 skewers alternating tomato, onion, bell pepper and tofu. Sprinkle with cumin and nutmeg. Cook under the broiler, on a barbeque or in the oven at 210°C 12 to 15 minutes based on how well done you want them.

Season with salt when done cooking.

Serve possibly drizzled with a little olive oil.

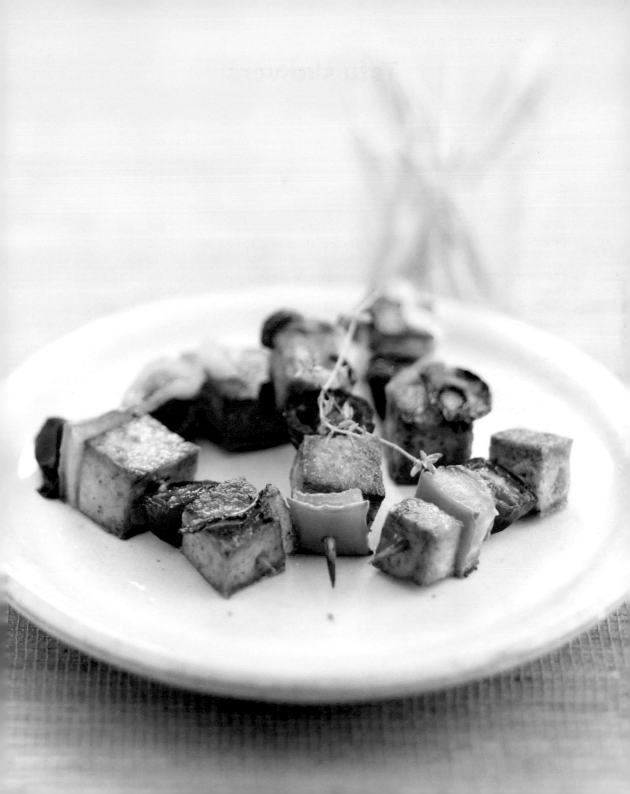

Vegetarian chili

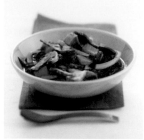

Serves 5

■ **Preparation time:**
20 minutes
■ **Cooking time:**
30 minutes

■ **Ingredients:**
> 1 green bell pepper
> 3 chopped onions
> 2 tablespoons of olive oil
> 2 crushed garlic cloves
> 1 can of kidney beans
(28oz - 800 g)
> 1 can of sliced
champignons (14oz - 400 g)
> 1 can of whole tomatoes
in their juice
> 9fl oz (25 cl) tomato puree
> 6 teaspoons of
tomato paste
> 1 teaspoon of cumin
> 3 teaspoons of chili powder
> 1 teaspoon of dry oregano
> 1 tablespoon of
unsweetened cocoa powder
> 1 pinch of Cayenne pepper
> 9fl oz (25 cl) red wine
> Salt and pepper

Open the bell pepper, deseed it and completely empty it. Using a large knife, cut the flesh into little pieces.

Sauté the chopped onions with olive oil in a frying pan. Halfway through cooking add the bell pepper and the garlic at the end of cooking.

Rinse the beans, drain the champignons in a strainer and remove the tomato juice.

In a skillet, pour in first the contents of the pan, then the beans, champignons and tomatoes. Mix, and season with salt and pepper. Add the tomato puree, tomato paste, cumin, chili powder, oregano, cocoa powder and Cayenne pepper. Pour in the wine until all the ingredients are covered. Let cook over a very low flame for 20 to 25 minutes. Adjust the seasoning. To make it spicier add a little chili and cumin.

Serve hot in soup bowls.

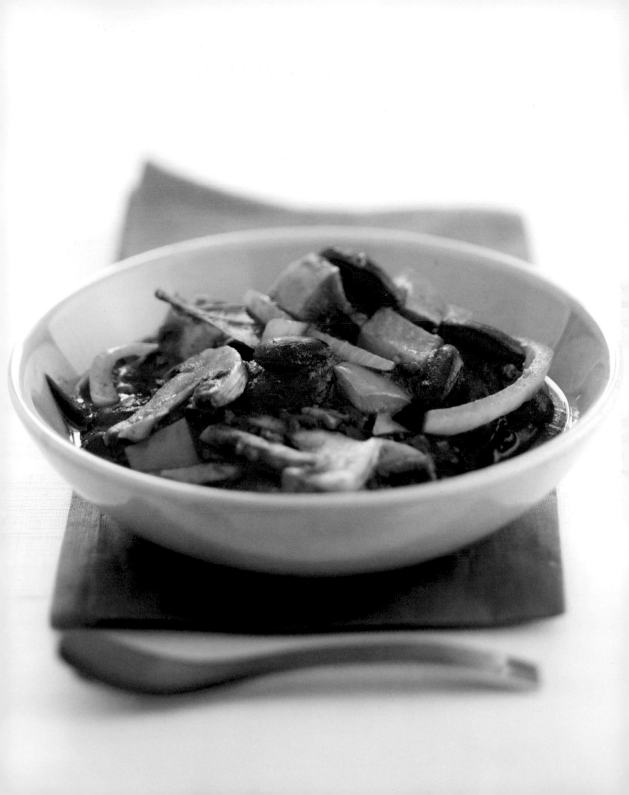

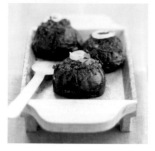

Vegetarian stuffed tomatoes

Serves 4

■ **Preparation time:**
15 minutes

■ **Cooking time:**
1h10 minutes

■ **Ingredients:**
> 8 tomatoes
> 2 onions
> 3 garlic cloves
> 1 large can of champignons
(around 14oz - 400 g drained)
> 9oz (250 g) of tofu
> Olive oil
> 2 tablespoons of
chopped parsley
> 3 egg whites
> 1 pinch of herbes
de Provence
> Salt and pepper

Open the tomatoes from the top and empty them using a small spoon. Save the flesh and drain it in a strainer. Deseed as much as possible. Turn the tomatoes over and let them drain.

Peel the onions and garlic. Chop the onions and mince the garlic. Drain the champignons and then cut them very finely. Chop the tofu.

Heat 1 tablespoon of olive oil in a large pan. Sauté the onions until they become very soft. Add the garlic at the end of cooking, Mix. Add the chopped tofu and continue cooking for 2 minutes while stirring. Add the champignons and parsley. Let cook for 1 to 2 minutes so that the moisture from the champignons evaporates. Add the tomato flesh last. Let cook for another 2 minutes while stirring with a spatula. Season with salt and pepper. Put in a salad bowl and let cool. Preheat the oven to 180°C.

Mix the egg whites into the previous mixture to make the stuffing.

Fill the empty tomatoes with the stuffing.

Place the stuffed tomatoes on a baking plate oiled with olive oil. Drizzle with olive oil and sprinkle herbes de Provence on top. Bake for around 1 hour.

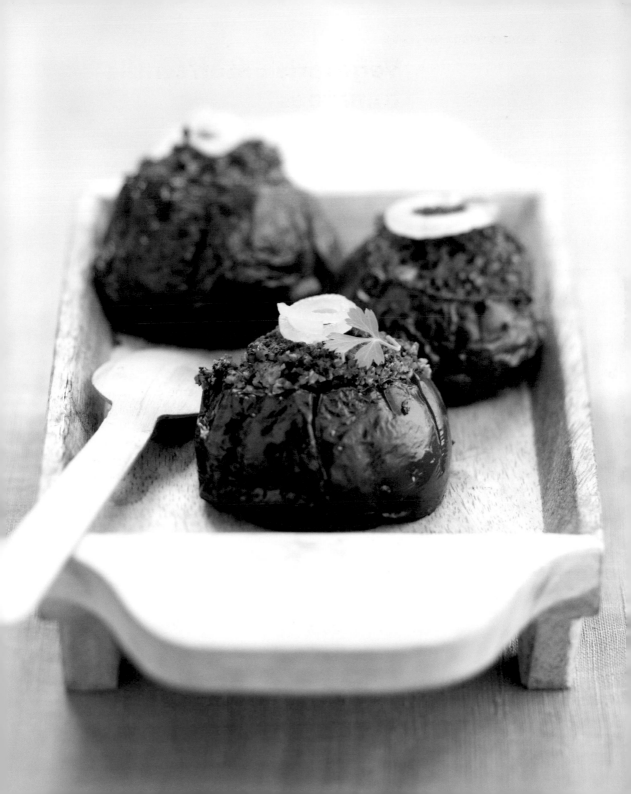

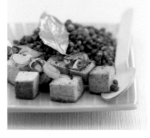

Tofu with green lentils

Serves 4

■ **Preparation time:**
5 minutes
■ **Cooking time:**
45 minutes

■ **Ingredients:**
> 9oz (250 g) Du Puy
green lentils
> Around 75 cl of
vegetable stock
> 1 bouquet garni
> 1 onion
> 1/2 tablespoon
of olive oil
> 14oz (400 g) of tofu
> 1 tablespoon of tamari
> Salt and pepper

In a skillet, put the lentils in three times their volume of vegetable stock. Add the bouquet garni. Let cook for 40 minute over a low flame. Lightly season with salt.

Peel and chop the onion. Brown with the olive oil in a frying pan over a low flame. Add the lentils.

When the lentils are cooked, season with salt and pepper.

Cut the tofu into 2 by 3 cm cubes.

In the pan where you cooked the onions, add olive oil if necessary and brown the tofu cubes over a high flame for 2 to 3 minutes. At the end of cooking pour in the tamari and deglaze with a spatula.

Serve the lentils in individual soup bowls. Put the tofu cubes on top with their sauce. Drizzle with olive oil if desired.

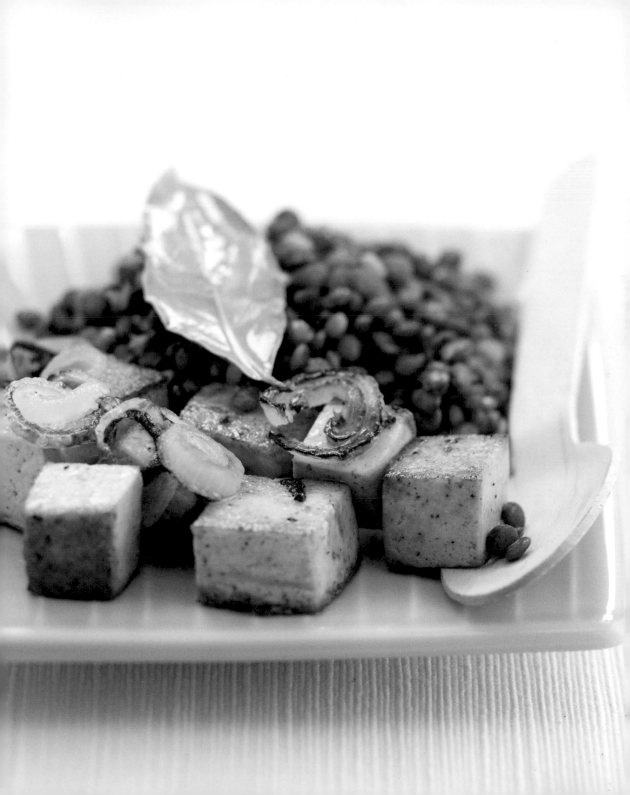

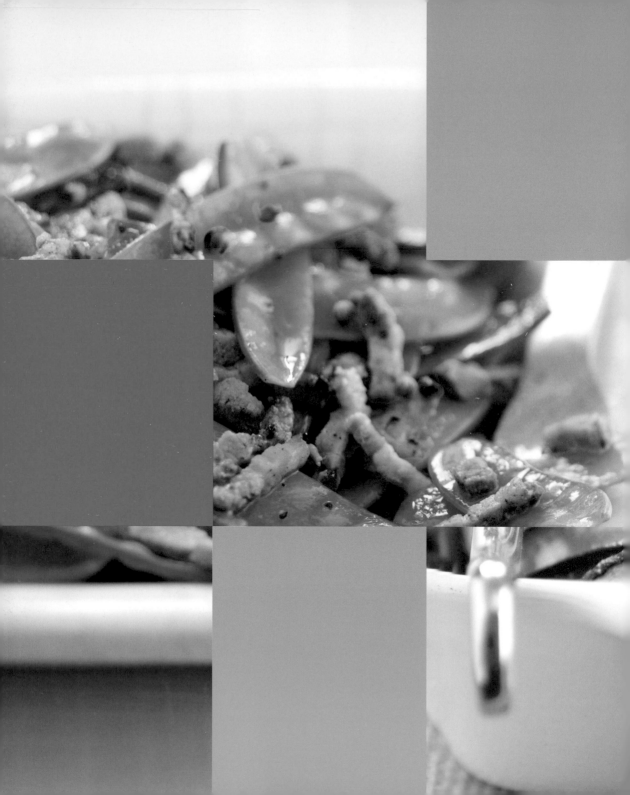

OTHERS

Endive with roquefort

Serves 4

■ **Preparation time:**
10 minutes

■ **Ingredients:**
> 5 sprigs of chive
> 5 radishes
> 5oz (150 g) of roquefort
> 3½ oz (100 g) of fresh goat cheese
> 2 endives
> Pepper

Chop the sprigs of chives and the radishes.

Mix the two cheeses, chopped chives and radishes with a fork. Season with pepper and mix.

Fill the endive leaves with the mixture.

Cucumbers with anchovies

Serves 4

■ **Preparation time:**
15 minutes
■ **Cooking time:**
6 minutes

■ **Ingredients:**
> 8 quail eggs
> 1 cucumber
> 1 can of anchovies
(4oz - 120 g)

Hard boil the quail eggs for 6 minutes in boiling water. Put them under cold water. Peel them and slice them in half.

Cut the cucumber in half lengthwise. Use a small spoon to empty it, save the flesh only. Cut it into pieces 3 cm long.

Put a toothpick in a half egg, then add a piece of cucumber, round side, so that it stays up. Thread the anchovy around, above the egg yolk.

Cubes of tuna omelet

Serves 4

■ **Preparation time:**
15 minutes
■ **Cooking time:**
40 minutes
■ **Refrigeration time:**
3 to 5 hours

■ **Ingredients:**
> 1 can of water
packed tuna (120 g)
> 12 black olives
> 1/2 whole yogurt
> 1 tablespoon of
tomato paste
> 3 eggs
> Olive oil for the dish
> Salt and pepper

Preheat the oven to 180 °C.

Drain the tuna and then mash it with a fork. Chop the black olives. Mix the yogurt and tomato paste.

Beat the eggs to make an omelet. Add the bits of tuna, black olives and tomato paste with yogurt. Season with salt and pepper.

Pour the mixture into an oiled baking dish. Bake in a double boiler for forty minutes. Let cool. Put in the refrigerator for 3 to 5 hours.

Cut the omelet into 2 cm squares and insert a wooden toothpick.

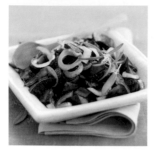

Montignac ratatouille

Serves 5

■ **Preparation time:**
30 minutes
■ **Cooking time:**
2 to 3 hours

■ **Ingredients:**
> 3 red bell peppers
> Olive oil
> 4 eggplants
> 5 medium size onions
> Herbes de Provence
> 9oz (250 g) tomato puree
> 3½ oz (100 g) tomato paste
> Salt and pepper

Preheat the oven to 130 °C.

Cut the bell peppers in half lengthwise. Empty them completely. Place the convex part up on a slightly oiled dripping pan. Bake for 2 to 2 and a half hour until the skin detaches.

Cut the eggplant into cubes of 2 to 3 cm and steam them 40 to 45 minutes. The pieces are cooked when they are very soft, even mushy, and they have turned brown. Place them in a large strainer and let them drain for at least 2 hours.

During this time, peel and chop the onions. Soften them with 3 tablespoons of olive oil over a low flame. Season with salt and pepper and add a few pinches of herbes de Provence.

Carefully peel the bell peppers with the tip of a knife. Cut the flesh into large pieces and set aside.

Put the drained eggplant in a large stockpot. Add the onions, bell peppers, tomato puree and tomato paste. Add 3 tablespoons of olive oil. Season with salt and pepper. Mix until it becomes uniform. Reheat over a very low flame or in a microwave oven.

Serve hot with a meat or fish or cold as an appetizer with a drizzle of olive oil and a few leaves of basil.

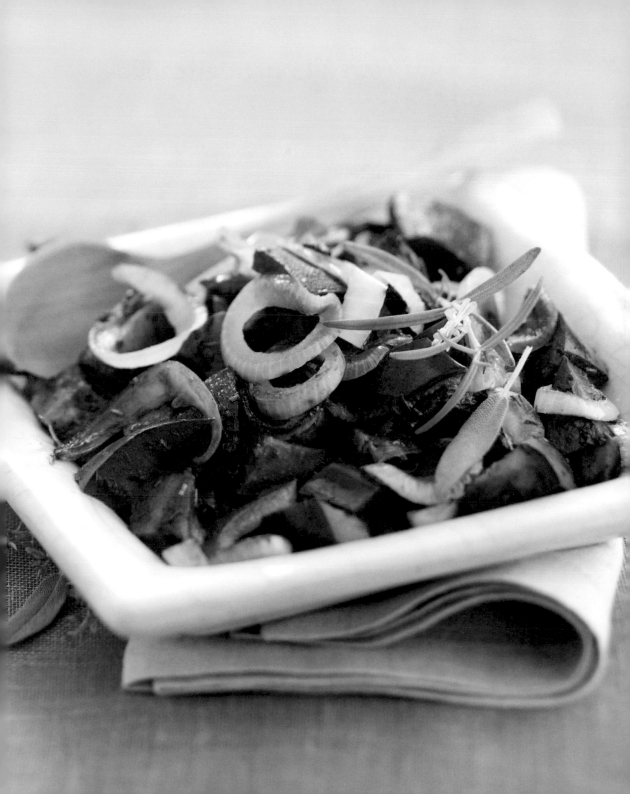

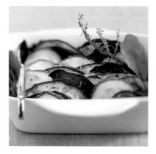

Tian à la provençale

Serves 4

■ **Preparation time:**
20 minutes
■ **Cooking time:**
1 hour

■ **Ingredients:**
> 4 eggplants
> 3 onions
> Olive oil
> 4 zucchini
> 8 tomatoes
> 3 tablespoons of
garlic powder
> 4 to 5 sprigs of parsley
> 2 teaspoons of
herbes de Provence
> Ten basil leaves
> Salt and pepper

Cut the eggplants in slices 1 cm thick. Cook them
15 minutes in a steamer and then let them drain.

Chop the onions and let them brown slightly in a frying
pan with 2 tablespoons of olive oil. Slice the zucchini
into rounds and sauté them in the frying pan with the
onions, adding a little oil.

Preheat the oven to 170 °C. Cut the tomatoes into
rounds and deseed them.

Oil a baking dish and alternate the eggplant, zucchini,
onion and tomatoes. End with the tomatoes.
Sprinkle the garlic powder, chopped parsley and herbes
de Provence. Season with salt and pepper and drizzle
with some olive oil. Bake for 40 to 45 minutes.

When serving, sprinkle with basil leaves and add a dash
of olive oil.

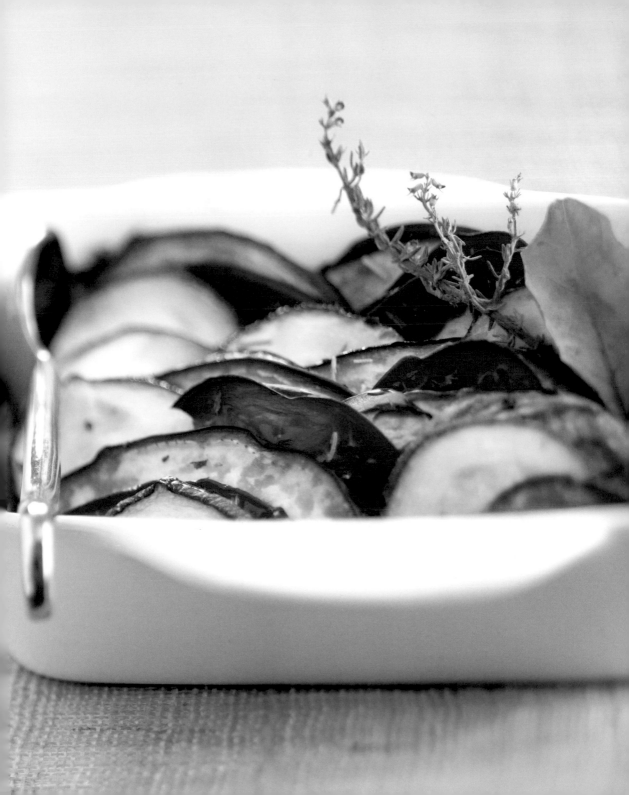

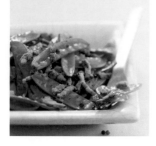

Snow peas with bacon

Serves 4

■ **Preparation time:**
10 minutes
■ **Cooking time:**
25 minutes

■ **Ingredients:**
> 1lb (500 g) snow peas
> 3 tablespoons of olive oil
> 3½ oz (100 g) natural
bacon cubes
> 3½ oz (100 g) smoked
bacon cubes
> Salt and pepper

Cut the ends off the snow peas. Put them under running water to wash them and then leave them to drain.

Heat a olive oil in a large pan. Pour in the snow peas. Cover. Let sweat over low flame. Stir every 2 minutes.

In another non-stick pan, sauté the bacon cubes without burning them.

When the peas are cooked (they should be tender), season with salt and pepper. Add the bacon cubes and stir. Continue cooking for 4 to 5 minutes uncovered and over a low flame, stirring regularly. Serve accompanied by a meat or an appetizer.

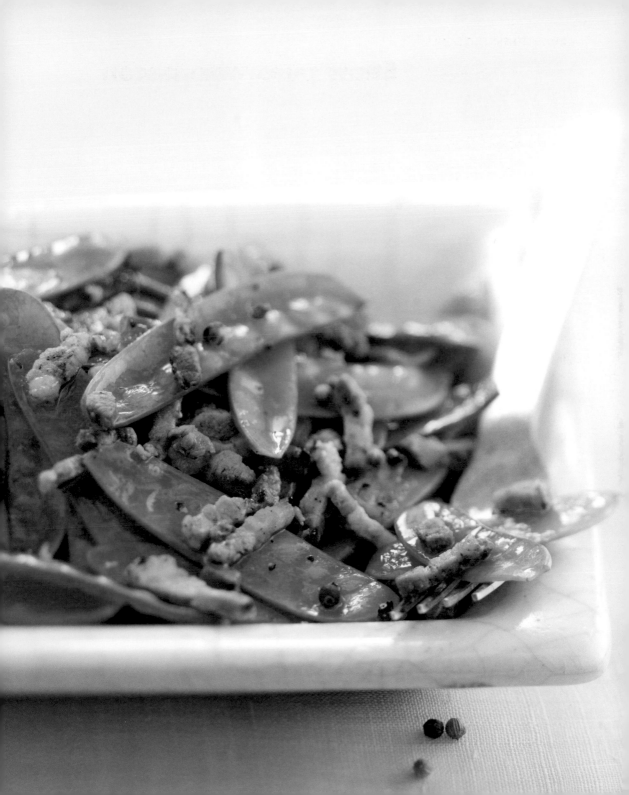

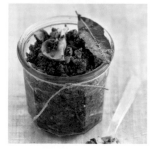

Meat sauce for pasta

Serves 4

■ **Preparation time:**
20 minutes
■ **Cooking time:**
20 minutes

■ **Ingredients:**
> 8 large tomatoes
> 3 and 1/2 soup
spoons of olive oil
> 5oz (150 g) julienne
natural bacon
> 14oz (400 g) of ground
beef
> 4 chopped onions
> 4 minced garlic cloves
> 3½ oz (100 g) of chopped
champignons
> 5 teaspoons
of tomato paste
> 5fl oz (15 cl) red wine
> 5fl oz (15 cl) of chicken
stock (fat-free extract)
> 1 pinch of nutmeg
> 1 bouquet garni (thyme,
bay leaf and parsley)
> 1 plain yogurt
> Salt and pepper

Drop the tomatoes into boiling water and cook for 40 seconds then under cold water. Peel them, seed them and crush them. Then let them drain.

Pour ½ tablespoon of olive oil into a large frying pan and slightly brown the bacon. Then add the ground beef, and separate it with a fork. Season and set aside.

In a skillet, pour in 3 tablespoons of olive oil and sauté the onion and then garlic over a low flame. Add the champignons. Then add the meat, the tomatoes, the tomato paste, red wine, chicken stock, pinch of nutmeg and bouquet garni. Mix it all and cook covered over a low flame for 15 minutes.

Add the yogurt and let the sauce reduce uncovered over a low flame, mixing regularly. Adjust the seasoning.

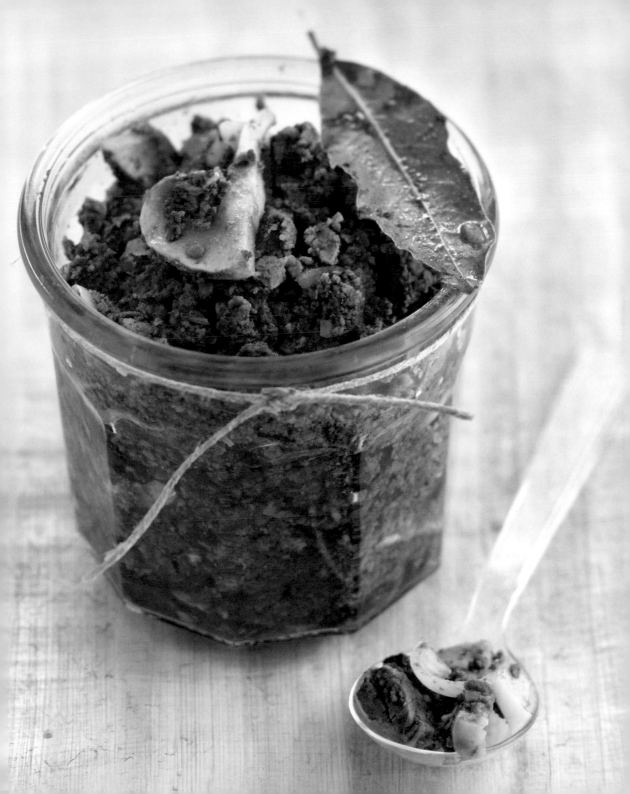

Basil tomato sauce

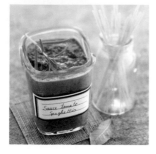

Serves 4

■ **Preparation time:**
5 minutes
■ **Cooking time:**
15 minutes

■ **Ingredients:**
> 14oz (400 g) tomato puree
> 3 tablespoons of
garlic powder
> 2 tablespoons of dry basil
> 1 tablespoon of
tomato extract
> 1 to fat-free yogurt
> 2 pinches of powdered
herbes de Provence
> A few fresh basil leaves
(for the garnish)
> Salt and pepper

In a skillet, pour in the contents of a can of tomato puree. Add the garlic powder, dry basil, tomato extract, fat-free yogurt and the herbes de Provence. Season with salt and pepper.

Cook in a double boiler for 15 minutes stirring constantly. Adjust the seasoning if necessary, decorate with basil and serve.

＊ This fat-free basil tomato sauce is perfect in phase I and can be used for spaghetti or rice for a carbohydrate-protein meal.

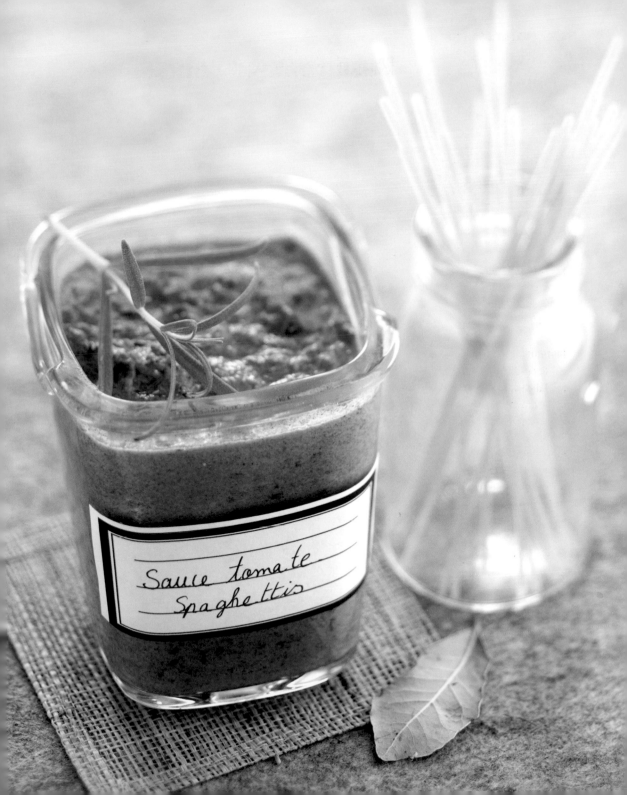

Sauce tomate
Spaghettis

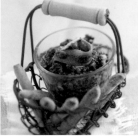

Tapenade provençale

Serves 4

■ **Preparation time:**
15 minutes

■ **Refrigeration time:**
2 to 3 hours

■ **Ingredients:**
> 4 garlic cloves
> 10 anchovy filets in olive oil
> 11oz (300 g) black olives
> 3½ oz (100 g) of capers
in vinegar
> 1/2 bunch of thyme
> Olive oil
> Pepper

Chop the garlic then crush in a mortar (or garlic press). Cut the anchovy filets into small pieces. Crush the anchovy with the garlic adding the oil from the anchovy jar.

Pit the black olives. Chop them finely with a knife.

Drain the capers and then cut them very finely.

Remove the thyme from the stalks and chop it finely.

Add the olives, capers and thyme to the mortar (or in a bowl). Crush to obtain a uniform past, drizzling olive oil. Season with pepper. Put the tapenade in a bowl and cover with plastic wrap. Let stand for 2 to 3 hours in the refrigerator.

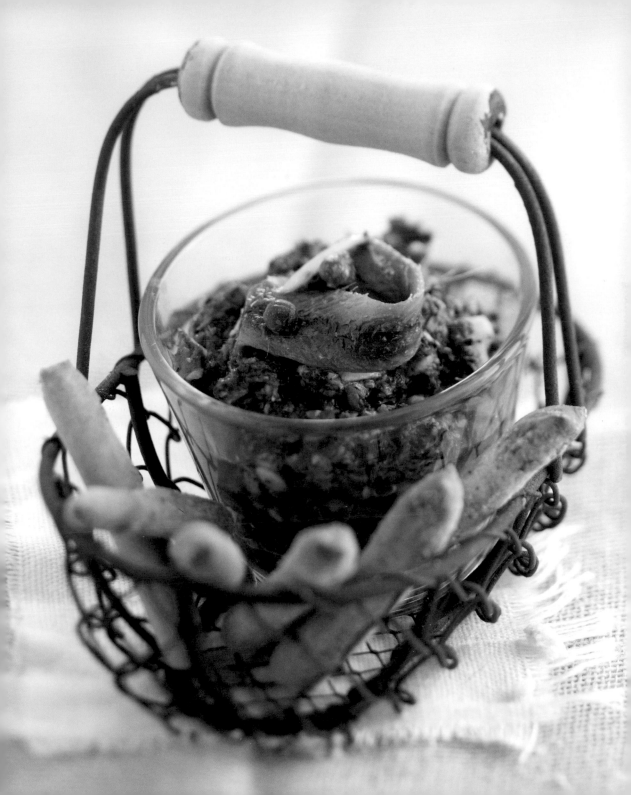

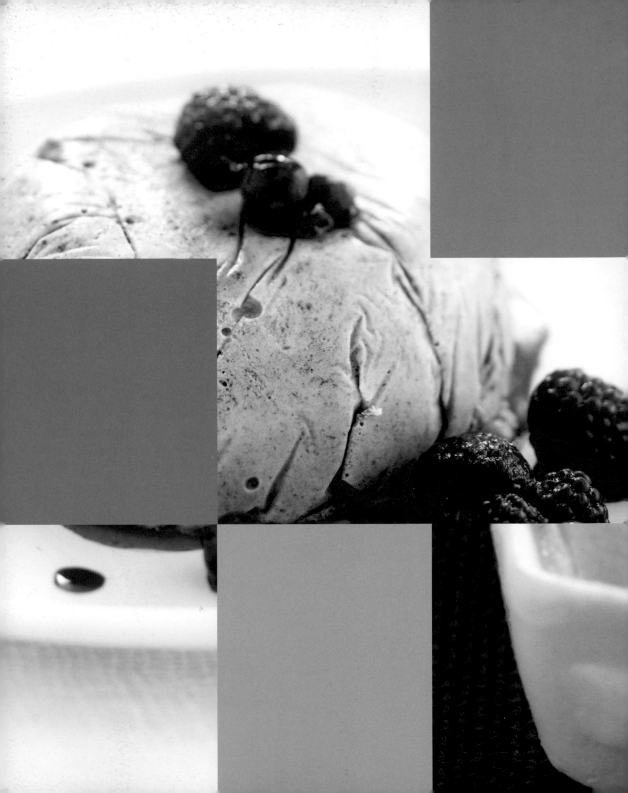

DESSERTS

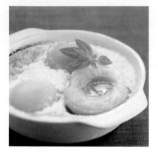

Flan with peaches

Serves 6

■ **Preparation time:**
15 minutes
■ **Cooking time:**
50 minutes

■ **Ingredients:**
> 2 cans of water packed peaches (2¼ lb - 1 kg each)
> 9fl oz (25 cl) whole liquid cream
> 8 eggs
> 2oz (50 g) fructose
> 4 cl of rum or cognac
> 3 teaspoons of vanilla extract

Preheat the oven to 170 °C.

Drain the peaches to completely eliminate any syrup from the can. Blend the peaches from one of the two cans (or chop them into very small pieces).
Put the others in the bottom of a layer cake pan; keep a few aside.

Whip the crème fraîche (for this to work well, the cream and the whisk need to be very cold).

Beat the eggs in a large bowl. Add the peach puree, fructose, rum (or cognac) and vanilla. Whisk. Add the whipped cream gently with a spatula. Put the mixture in the pan on top of the peaches. Arrange the remaining peaches on top. Bake 45 to 50 minutes.

Check if cooked by inserting the tip of a knife in the cake. If the blade comes out dry, it is done.

Let it cool before serving.

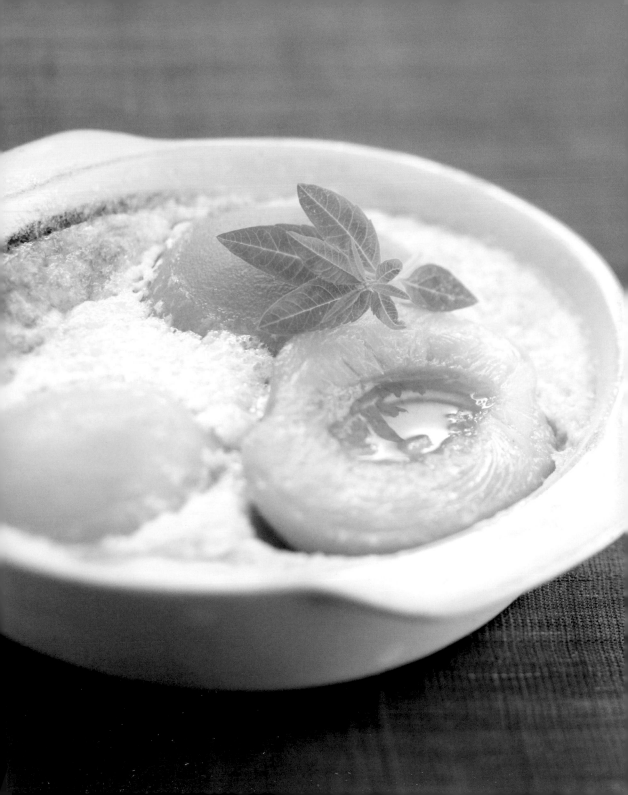

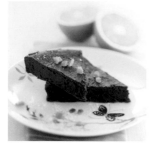

Bitter chocolate fondant

Serves 4

■ **Preparation time:**
25 minutes
■ **Cooking time:**
15 minutes

■ **Ingredients:**
> 2 teaspoons of
instant coffee
> 11oz (300 g) of dark bitter
chocolate with 70% cocoa
> 2fl oz (5 cl) rum
> 1 untreated orange
> 6 large fresh eggs (organic)
> 1 pinch of salt

Make a small cup of strong coffee with the instant coffee.

In a skillet, place the chocolate cut into pieces, and add the coffee and rum. Heat in a double boiler. Stir with a wooden spoon to mix well. As soon as the chocolate has the consistency of a thick, smooth cream, remove the skillet from the double boiler.

Grate the orange zest, only using the surface part of the peel. Put half the zest in the chocolate and mix. Separate the eggs. Whip the whites until stiff (after having added 1 pinch of salt). Preheat the oven to 250 °C.

Pour the melted chocolate into a salad bowl with the yolks. Mix until obtaining a uniform cream. Fold the whites into this mixture with a rubber spatula until no parts of the white remain. Make sure that no unmixed chocolate has fallen into the bottom of the bowl.

Line a non-stick mold with greaseproof paper. Pour in the mixture. Sprinkle the rest of the zest on it. Put it in the oven after making sure it is hot. Bake only 8 minutes. Take it out of the oven, even if you think it is not cooked enough. Let cool.

Serve as is or with a thin custard sauce.

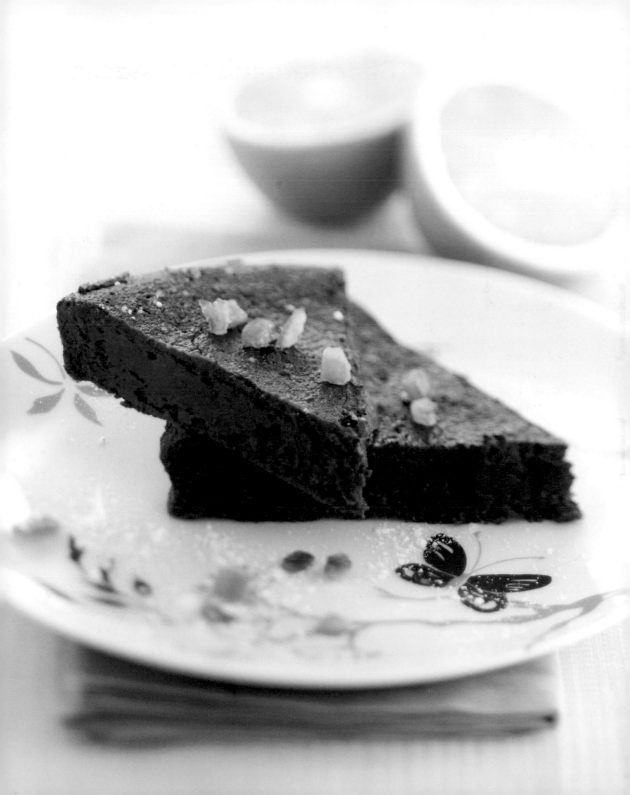

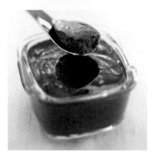

Chocolate mousse

Serves 4

★ To make the day before

■ **Preparation time:**
25 minutes
■ **Refrigeration time:**
at least 6 hours
■ **Cooking time:**
10 minutes

■ **Ingredients:**
> 2 teaspoons of
instant coffee
> 11oz (300 g) of dark bitter
chocolate with 70% cocoa
> 2fl oz (5 cl) rum
> 1 untreated orange
> 6 large fresh eggs (organic)
> 1 pinch of salt

Make a small cup of strong coffee with the instant coffee.

In a double boiler, melt the chocolate, coffee and rum. Stir with a wooden spoon to mix well. As soon as the chocolate has the consistency of a thick, smooth cream, remove the skillet from the double boiler.

Grate the orange zest, only using the surface part of the peel. Put half the zest in the chocolate and mix.

Separate the eggs and put the yolks in a large salad bowl. Whip the whites until stiff (after having added 1 pinch of salt).

Pour the melted chocolate into a salad bowl with the yolks. Mix until obtaining a uniform cream. Fold the whites into this mixture with a rubber spatula until no parts of the white remain. Make sure that no unmixed chocolate has fallen into the bottom of the bowl.

Keep the mousse in the salad bowl – in this case, carefully dry the edges -, pour it into a compote dish or fill individual ramekins. Sprinkle with the rest of the orange zest and chill for at least 6 hours.

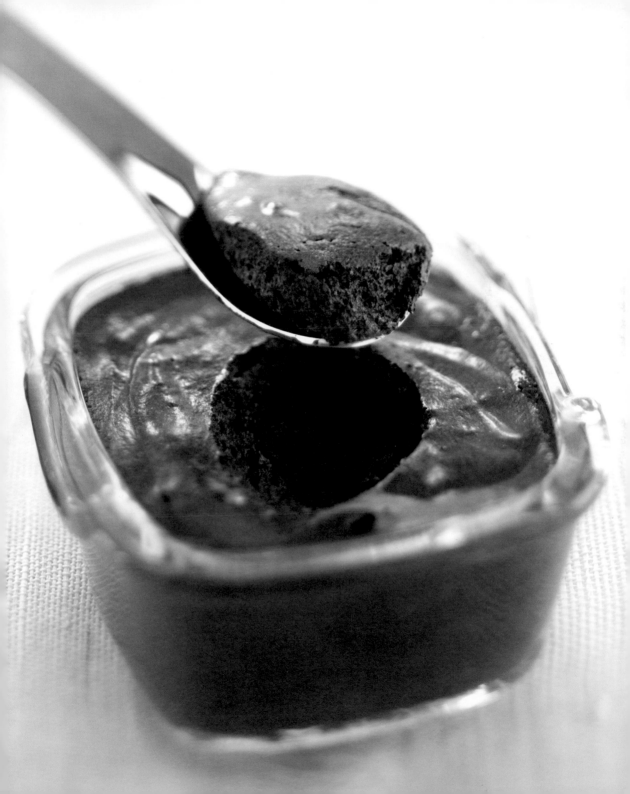

Bavarois with berries

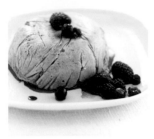

Serves 4

★ To make the day before

■ **Preparation time:**
20 minutes
■ **Cooking time:**
5 minutes
■ **Refrigeration time:**
12 hours

■ **Ingredients:**
> 1oz (20 g) of gelatin leaves
> 3½ oz (100 g) fructose
> 21oz (600 g) of berries
(raspberries, strawberries,
blackcurrants, blueberries)
> 9fl oz (25 cl) crème fraîche
> 1 small bunch of mint
(for the garnish)

Put the gelatin in a bowl of cold water.

Heat 6 cl of water in a pan with the fructose. Let cook over a low flame until obtaining a syrupy liquid.

Press the gelatin by hand to wring it out. Add it to the fructose syrup. Let it melt while mixing. Pour it into a cup and set aside.

After washing and preparing the fruit, blend them to reduce them to a puree. Add the syrup.

Whip the crème fraîche until stiff (for this to work well, the cream and the whisk need to be very cold).

Add the pureed fruit in the syrup to the whipped cream and mix gently.

Pour this mixture into a non-stick Charlotte pan. Let it set in the refrigerator overnight. Unmold before serving and garnish with a few leaves of mint.

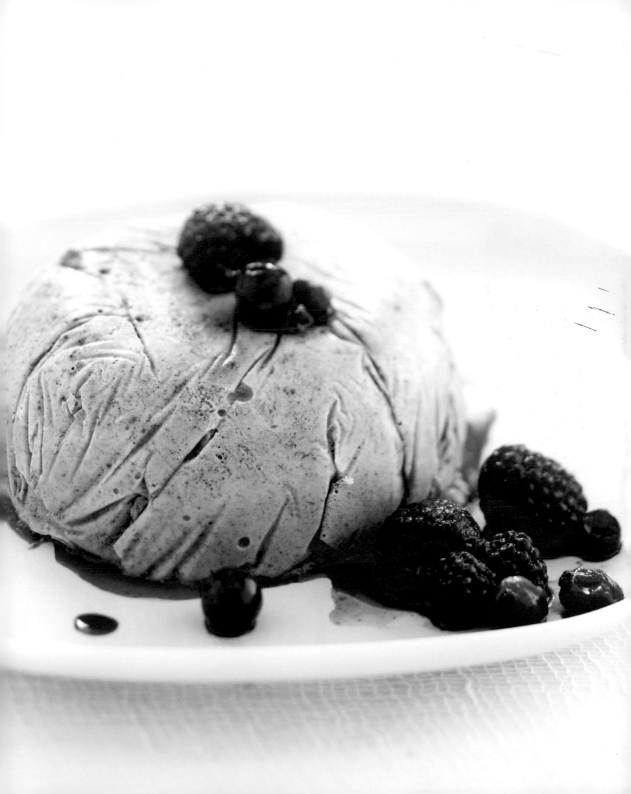

Corsican fresh cheese cake

Serves 4

■ **Preparation time:**
25 minutes
■ **Cooking time:**
40 minutes

■ **Ingredients:**
> 9oz (250 g) fresh Corsican
cheese – brocciu
(or other fresh goat
or ewe cheese)
> 1 untreated lemon
> 3 eggs
> 2oz (60 g) fructose
> 1 pinch of salt
> Olive oil for the mold

Preheat the oven to 180°C.

Drain the cheese in a sieve.

Remove 4 thin zests from the lemon 5 to 6 cm long.
Drop them into a small pot of boiling water and blanche
for 3 minutes. Drain and then chop finely.

Separate the whites from the yolks and put them in
separate bowls. Add the fructose to the yolks. Whisk until
obtaining a creamy mixture. Mash the cheese with a
fork in a plate. Add it to the yolks and add the chopped
lemon zest. Stir to obtain a uniform mixture.

Add the salt to the egg whites and whip them with an
electric mixer until they are stiff. Gently add the egg
whites to the mixture with a spatula.

Oil the cake pan with the olive oil. Pour the mixture into
the cake pan. Bake for 35 minutes. Check the cooking
by inserting a sharp knife : the blade should be dry.
Let it cool slightly before removing from the cake pan.

Compote à l'ancienne

Serves 4

■ **Preparation time:**
20 minutes
■ **Soaking time:**
1 hour
■ **Cooking time:**
6 minutes

■ **Ingredients:**
> 2oz (50 g) pitted prunes
> 3 untreated oranges
> 4 apricots
> 2 yellow peaches
> 7oz (200 g) red grapes
> 7oz (200 g) green grapes
> 4fl oz (10 cl) sweet wine
(monbazillac)
> 2oz (40 g) fructose
> 1/4 tablespoon of
cinnamon powder
> 2oz (40 g) plain Greek
yogurt
> 2oz (40 g) of chopped
pistachios (for the garnish)

Let the prunes soak in a bowl of water for at least 1 hour. Drain them.

With a zest knife, remove thin zests from an orange. Peel 1 orange and remove the quarters eliminating all their peel. Juice the other two oranges.

Wash the apricots. Cut them in half and remove the pit. Drop the peaches into boiling water for a few seconds. Peel them, remove the pit and cut into slices. Rinse the grapes and dry them.

Put the peaches, apricots, grapes, prunes and orange quarters into a pan. Add the orange juice, sweet wine, fructose and cinnamon. Bring to a boil, cover and let simmer for 5 minutes.

Remove all the fruit with a skimmer and reduce the juice to a syrup. Mix the syrup and yogurt in a bowl.

Divide the compote into four soup plates. Coat with yogurt.

Garnish with orange zest and chopped pistachios.

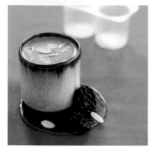

Prune mousse

Serves 4

■ **Preparation time:**
15 minutes
■ **Soaking time:**
1 hour
■ **Refrigeration time:**
2 hours

■ **Ingredients:**
> 1 teabag
> 7oz (200 g) pitted prunes
> 2fl oz (5 cl) cognac
> 8 petits-suisses or 14oz
(400 g) of fresh goat cheese
> 4fl oz (10 cl) low-fat liquid
crème fraîche
> 1 teaspoon of natural
vanilla extract
> 1¾ oz (30 g) fructose
> 2oz (50 g) crushed
almonds
> 1 untreated orange
(for the garnish)

Make a cup of strong tea. Put the prunes in a bowl and pour in the tea and cognac. Let steep for around 1 hour.

Drain the prunes. Mix them in a mixer to make a puree.

Put the petits-suisses (or goat cheese) in a bowl. Add the liquid cream, vanilla extract and fructose. Whisk until this mixture becomes slightly frothy. Add the prune puree and crushed almonds. Mix well.

Pour the mousse into small dishes and chill for 2 hours.

Garnish with orange zest.

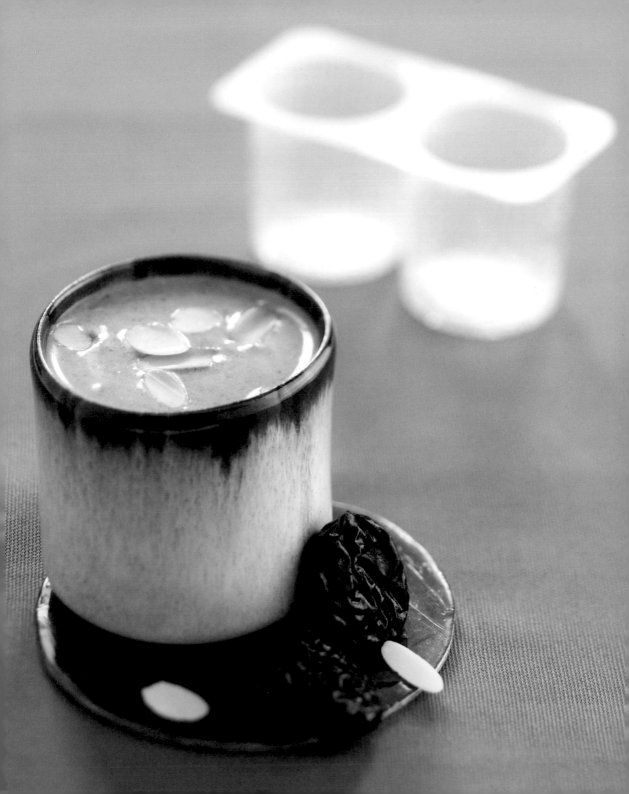

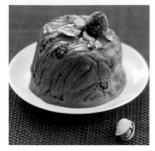

Parfait with chocolate, raspberries and pistachios

Serves 4

■ **Preparation time:**
30 minutes
■ **Cooking time:**
20 minutes
■ **Freezing time:**
4 hours

■ **Ingredients:**
For the fruit garnish
> 2oz (50 g) fructose
> 9oz (250 g) fresh
raspberries
> 2oz (50 g) of shelled pista-
chios crushed and grilled
> 2 teaspoons of natural
vanilla extract

■ **For the chocolate parfait
mousse**
> 7oz (200 g) of dark bitter
chocolate with more
than 70% cocoa
> 1½ oz (30 g) fructose
> 2fl oz (5 cl) rum
> 4 egg yolks
> 1oz (25 g) of liquid
crème fraîche (with 35% fat
content)

Pour 2oz (50 g) of fructose and 6 cl of water into a pot. Bring to a boil until the syrup thickens. Add the rasp-berries, pistachios and vanilla. Heat for a little more than 5 minutes and then remove from the burner. Let cool and then chill.

Break the chocolate up into small pieces in a large bowl. Put it on top of a pan of simmering water and melt the chocolate.

Pour 30 g of fructose and then rum into a pan.
Heat until obtaining a thick syrup.

During this time, whisk the yolks until they turn white. Continue whisking while pouring in the rum syrup in a stream. Whisk very quickly for 4 to 5 minutes. Add the melted chocolate.

Whip the crème fraîche then gently add it to the previous mixture with a spatula. Add the fruit and stir.

Pour it all into a mold covered with greaseproof paper. Fold the paper over the mixture and freeze for at least 4 hours.

To unmold, remove the greaseproof paper and cut the parfait into slices.

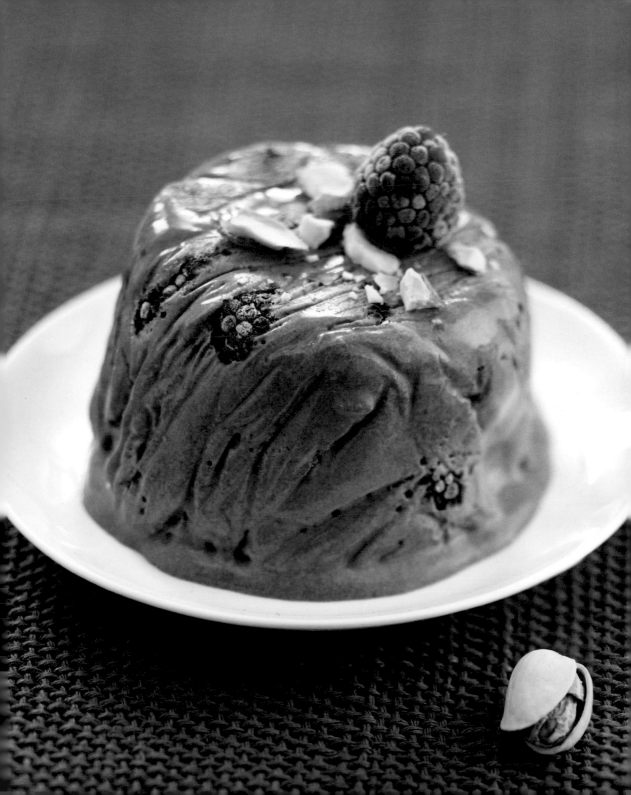

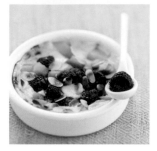

Fruit zabaglione with almonds

Serves 5

■ **Preparation time:**
30 minutes

■ **Cooking time:**
12 minutes

■ **Ingredients:**
> 4 yellow peaches
> 1lb (500 g) strawberries
> 8 apricots
> 9oz (250 g) raspberries
(keep 4 for garnishing)
> 5 egg yolks
> 2oz (50 g) fructose
> 2fl oz (5 cl) cognac
> 3½ oz (100 g) crème
fraîche
> 2oz (50 g) almond powder
> 3 tablespoons
flakes almonds
> Olive oil for the molds

Boil the peaches for a few seconds. Peel them and remove the pits. Cut them into large chunks. Remove the peduncle from the strawberries and cut them into pieces (keep a few for the garnish). Open the apricots, remove the pits and cut into large rounds.
Rinse the raspberries.

Oil four individual baking dishes and divide the fruit into them.

Heat water in a large pan. Place the yolks in a bowl which can withstand heat. Add 30 g of fructose and the cognac. Whisk until this mixture turns white. Put the bowl in the pan with boiling water. Continue to whisk to obtain a thick cream. Remove from the double boiler and add the crème fraîche and almond powder while whisking.

Cover the fruit with this mixture. Turn on the broiler.

Sprinkle the surface of the cream with the remaining fructose. Sprinkle with the almond flakes. Put the baking dishes as close as possible to the broiler. Let them brown for around 2 to 3 minutes, watching to take them out on time.

Garnish with strawberries and raspberries, serve immediately.

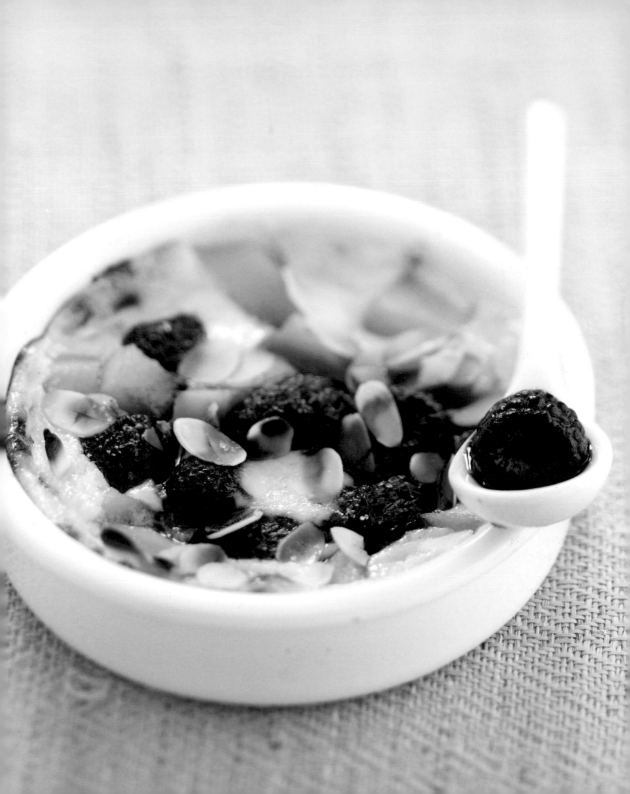

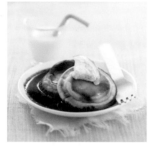

Goat cheese cake

Serves 4

■ **Preparation time:**
15 minutes
■ **Cooking time:**
40 minutes

■ **Ingredients:**
> 1 untreated lemon
> 3 eggs + 1 yolk
> 2½ oz (70 g) fructose
> 9oz (250 g) of fresh goat cheese
> 3½ oz (100 g) crème fraîche
> 2oz (50 g) plain thick yogurt
> 1 teaspoon of natural vanilla extract
> Olive oil for the mold

Grate the lemon zests.

Separate the whites from the yolks and whip the whites until stiff.

Oil a layer cake pan. Preheat the oven to 160 °C.

In a salad bowl, whisk the 4 yolks and fructose until the mixture turns white. Add the fresh goat cheese, crème fraîche, yogurt, lemon zests and vanilla. Mix well.

Gently fold in the stiff egg whites with a spatula.

Pour into the cake pan. Bake 35 to 40 minutes.

Serve warm or cold with a raspberry coulis.

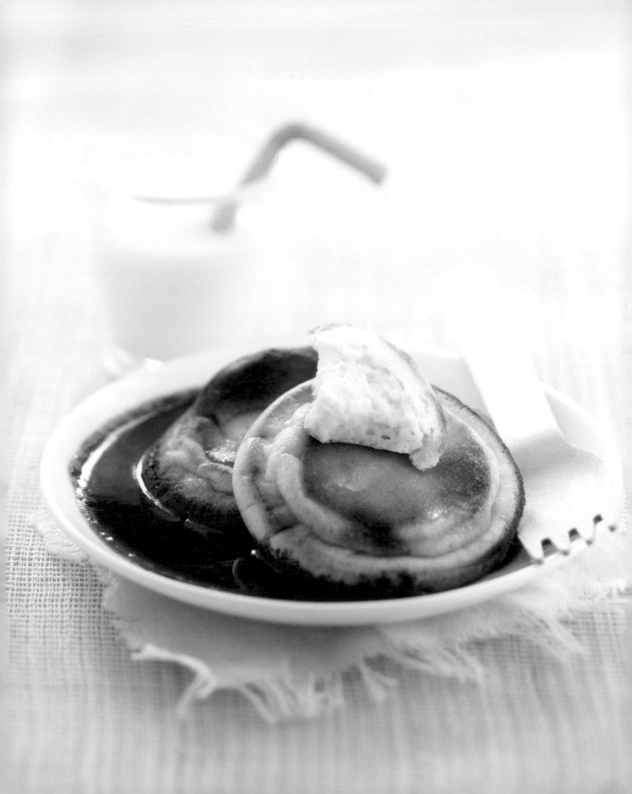

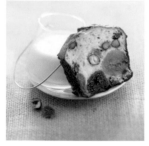

Three fruit cake

Serves 4

■ **Preparation time:**
1 hour
■ **Soaking time:**
1 hour
■ **Cooking time:**
45 minutes

■ **Ingredients:**
> 11oz (300 g) dried figs
> 7oz (200 g) pitted prunes
> 7oz (200 g) dried apricots
> 4fl oz (10 cl) rum
> 50 whole hazelnuts
> 2oz (50 g) whole almonds
> 3½ oz (100 g) almond
powder
> 2oz (50 g) hazelnut powder
> 1/2 teaspoon of cinnamon
> 9fl oz (25 cl) low-fat
crème fraîche
> 3 eggs + 1 egg white
> Olive oil for the mold

Cut the figs, prunes and apricots into small pieces and marinate them in the rum for an hour.

Preheat the oven to 160 °C.

Chop the hazelnuts and almonds coarsely. Put them in a salad bowl then add the almond and hazelnut powders, cinnamon and crème fraîche. Mix with a spatula.

Whisk the eggs with the white and pour into the salad bowl. Add the marinated fruit without the juice and mix everything.

Oil a cake pan. Pour all the mixture into the cake pan. Bake for around 45 minutes. Let it cool slightly before removing from the cake pan.

✱ This cake can be eaten plain, with a vanilla flavored thin custard or served with fresh cheese.

✱ This cake is ideal for an athlete's breakfast.

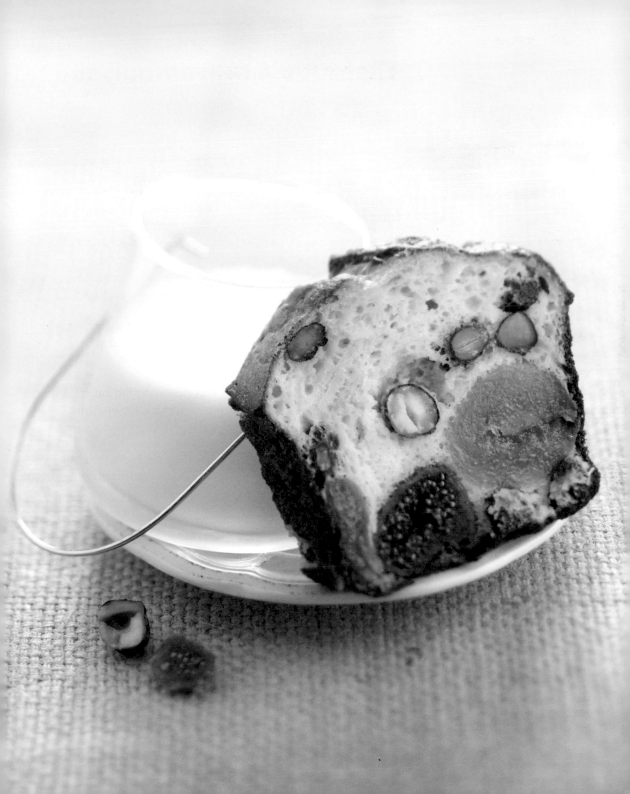

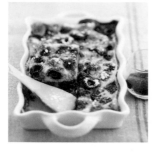

Clafoutis aux framboises

Serves 4

■ **Preparation time:**
15 minutes
■ **Cooking time:**
30 minutes

■ **Ingredients:**
> 3 eggs
> 4oz (125 g) low-fat
crème fraîche
> 1½ oz (30 g) fructose
(+ a little for the pan)
> 2fl oz (5 cl) raspberry
brandy (rum or cognac
or even ½ teaspoon of
natural vanilla extract)
> 11oz (300 g) raspberries
> Olive oil for the pan

Preheat the oven to 180 °C.

Break the eggs in a salad bowl. Add the cream and fructose. Beat until the mixture becomes very uniform. Pour in the raspberry brandy and mix again.

Oil a baking dish and lightly sprinkle its sides with fructose.

Put the raspberries on the bottom of the pan and cover with the batter.

Bake 25 to 30 minutes.

Serve warm or cold possibly with a fructose icing.

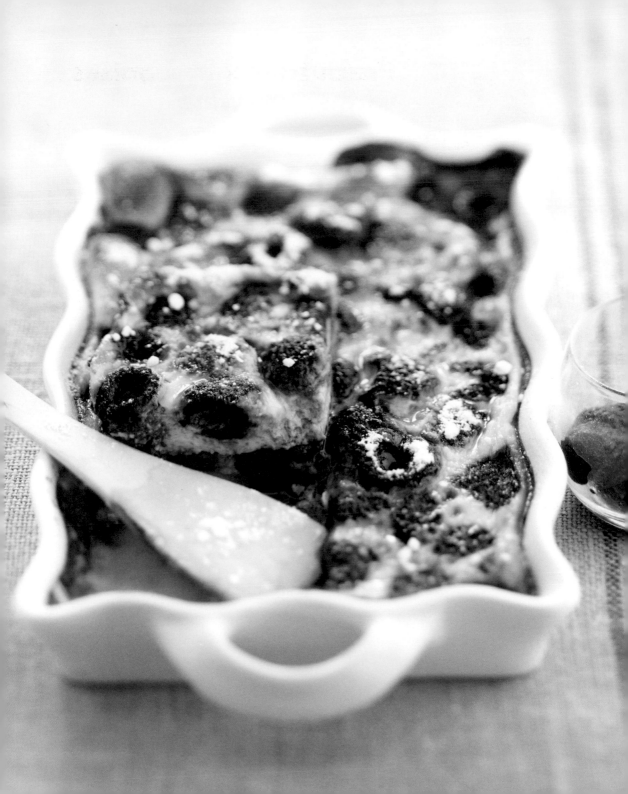

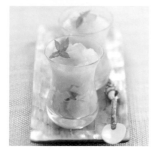

Peach soup
with sweet wine

Serves 4

★ To make the day before

■ **Preparation time:**
15 minutes
■ **Refrigeration time:**
12 hours

■ **Ingredients:**
> 4 large yellow peaches
> 2 large white peaches
> 1 bunch of fresh mint
> 1 glass of monbazillac,
barsac or pacherenc, chilled
> 4 teaspoons of fructose

Drop the peaches into boiling water. Put them in cold water and then peel. Chill the yellow peaches.

Cut the white peaches into pieces and mix them with a dozen leaves of fresh mint. Add the glass of sweet wine and fructose. Put it through a sieve to remove some of the moisture. Put the puree in a bowl and chill overnight.

Cut the yellow peaches into cubes and place them in the bottom of bell-shaped glasses. Pour over the peach soup prepared to night before and garnish with fresh mint.

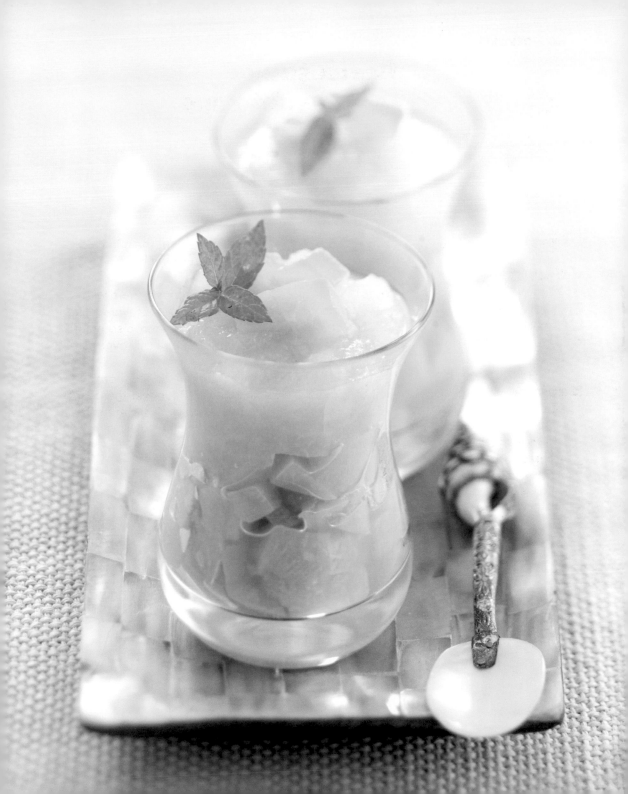

Apricot cake

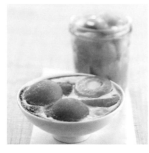

Serves 4

■ **Preparation time:**
15 minutes
■ **Cooking time:**
50 minutes

■ **Ingredients:**
> 21oz (600 g) of apricots
> 4 eggs + 1 yolk
> 2½ oz (70 g) fructose
> 9fl oz (25 cl) low-fat
crème fraîche
> Olive oil for the pan

Preheat the oven to 170 °C. Oil a baking dish (preferably a round non-stick metallic pan)

Cut two thirds of the apricots in half to remove the pit. Put the apricot halves on the bottom of the pan with the convex side down. Bake for 10 minutes.

Cut the rest of the apricots into pieces. Mix them in a mixer to make a puree.

Beat the eggs and the white in a bowl. Add the fructose, crème fraîche, apricot puree and apricot cooking juice from the oven. Mix well.

Pour it all on the pre-cooked apricots still on the bottom of the pan.

Bake 35 to 40 minutes. Check the cooking by inserting a blade of a sharp knife: if the blade comes out dry, the cake is done.

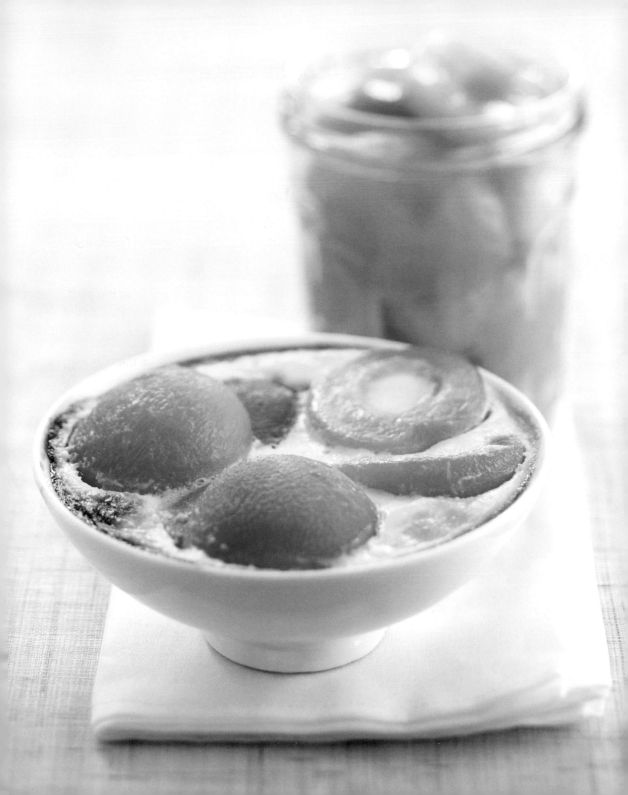

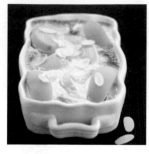

Nectarine cake with almonds

Serves 4

■ **Preparation time:**
15 minutes
■ **Cooking time:**
43 minutes

■ **Ingredients:**
> 5 white nectarines
> 5 tablespoons of fructose
> 5 eggs
> 4oz (125 g) almond
powder
> 1 thick yogurt
(made with whole milk)
> 1/2 teaspoon of natural
vanilla extract
> 2oz (40 g) almond flakes

Preheat the oven to 170 °C.

Open the nectarines and remove the pits. Cut them into 6 sections. Place them higgledy-piggledy in a baking pan suitable for a microwave oven. Sprinkle with 1 table-spoon of fructose. Mix. Precook for 3 minutes in the microwave.

Beat the eggs in a bowl. Add the almond powder, yogurt, 4 tablespoons of fructose and vanilla. Whisk.

Pour it on the nectarines in the baking pan. Distribute the almond flakes on top. Bake for 40 minutes.

Five minutes before removing the pan fro the oven, turn on the broiler to brown the almonds.

Let it cool before serving.

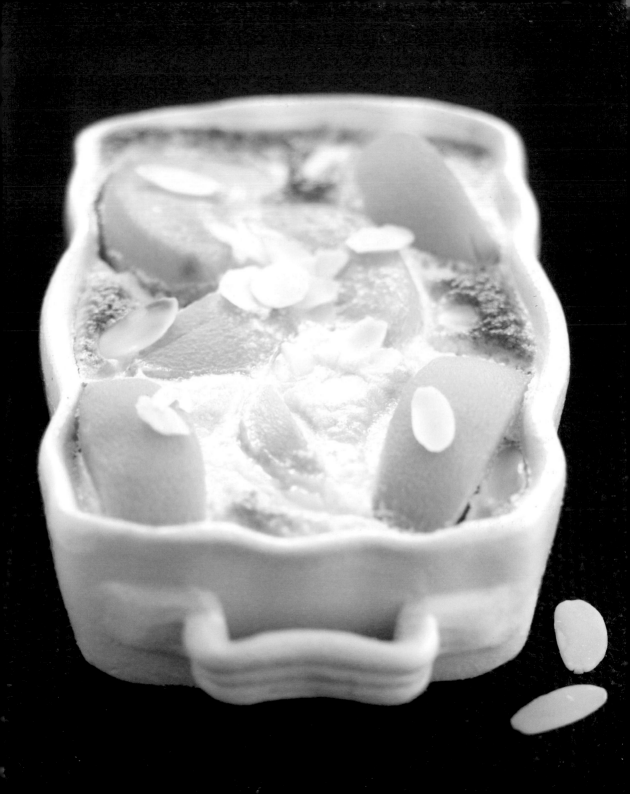

Index by products

Michel Montignac© products

More than 180 products for eating healthy every day and pleasing your taste buds. Michel Montignac has created an exclusive range of food products, especially conceived for following his method. They are all rich in fiber, with no added sugar, created from organic whole-wheat flour and have in common a low glycemic index. They also do not contain artificial colors, additives or modified starches.
They include 100% fruit specialties, crackers and toast, cookies and chocolate with a high cocoa content (70% and 85%), pasta, compotes and coulis.
Michel Montignac products are sold in more than 1,000 stores in France, particularly gourmet shops, health food stores and stores selling diet products. But they can also be found abroad, in most European countries.

You can find all the information for buying these products on
www.montignac-shop.com

The official website:
www.montignac.com

Coaching online:
www.methode-montignac.com

Other books by Michel Montignac

Eat Yourself Slim, Alpen, 2010.
The Montignac Diet Cookbook, Alpen, 2010.
Glycemic Index Diet, Alpen, 2010.